"This is a unique resource that takes you to the inner response and thoughts of women in turmoil. Both the women considering abortion and those seeking a way to help them are looking for answers. For those confronted with 'What do I do?' and those wondering 'What do I say?' this book has answers. This resource reflects the understanding of the author and assists the reader in what they can say and do to help others. It combines the findings of research with the practical, and the writing of this author reflects his depth of knowledge and ability to take this information he has gathered and present it in a helpful manner. Anyone working in this field will be appreciative of this new resource."

—Dr. H. Norman Wright
Licensed Marriage Child Family Therapist
Certified Trauma Specialist,
Traumatologist, Board Certified in Bereavement Trauma
Trainer and Board Member of Victim Relief Ministries
Author of *The Complete Guide to Crisis & Trauma Counseling*

"A great training tool for the person wanting to be an effective crisis intervention counselor! 'Where do I start? I'm afraid I'll do it wrong.' *Pregnancy Crisis Intervention* can calm their fears, give basic understanding of unexpected pregnancy issues, and provide counselor tools to launch them into the role of encourager and helper. While more training will be needed to fine-tune their skills, John Ensor's encouragement to build a relationship bridge *first* is an invaluable place to begin."

—Bobbie Meyer, State Director
Carolina Pregnancy Care Fellowship
Charlotte, North Carolina

"John Ensor is a visionary, and this book is the perfect complement to our onsite training program. I've read and reread the chapters, and I'm learning and enjoying his wise and excellent perspective."

—Sylvia Johnson-Matthews
Executive Director, Houston Pregnancy Help Centers

"John Ensor truly understands the intervention process for helping women and men who are going through this difficult time. Our centers will be using *Pregnancy Crisis Intervention* as a training tool for all who have a calling to counsel."

—Sol Pitchon, President   irector
                                   Florida

D0684248

"Pregnancy Crisis Intervention is a good read—presenting valuable material in a very user-friendly format. It is now required reading for all new staff and volunteers at our center!"

—**Kim H. Bennett, RN, BS, CCE**
· **Program Director, AlphaCare, Philadelphia**

"With years of experience, John Ensor presents clear, concise insights for helping women in crisis pregnancies. His book provides valuable guidance not only for beginners but also for the experienced counselor. I highly recommend *Pregnancy Crisis Intervention* as a valuable resource for every pregnancy help organization."

—**Marianne Casagrande, New Hope Clinic, Butte, Montana**

"Pregnancy Crisis Intervention is a valuable and practical tool for providing authentic help to women during an overwhelming time in their life. This is just what you need to love well and empower women to make healthy decisions for themselves and their baby."

—**Vicky Botsford Mathews, President, LifeSteward Ministries**
Executive Director, Choices Women's Clinic, Orlando

"With gracious wisdom and crystal clarity, John Ensor provides the solid research, biblically based principles, and practical steps every Christian needs to confidently speak the truth in love when helping a woman in a pregnancy crisis. An invaluable resource for pregnancy help organizations and for anyone facing this critical conversation!"

—**Susanne Maynes, Author,**
Unleashing Your Courageous Compassion:
40 Reflections on Rescuing the Unborn

"This much-needed book offers great insight and methods on how to deal with the unique issues associated with pregnancy crisis intervention. Through decades of experience and thorough research, John Ensor has created the most comprehensive resource for anyone ministering to women in pregnancy crisis. This book is now required reading in the training of our patient advocates and client care/medical staff."

—**Peggy Benicke, Executive Director**
Robbinsdale Women's Center, Minneapolis

"An insightful and practical guide! You'll learn as a first responder how to go from a crisis intervention transaction to a relational transformation."

—**Amy Scheuring, Women's Choice Network, Pittsburgh**

Pregnancy Crisis
INTERVENTION

Pregnancy Crisis
INTERVENTION

What to Do and Say When It Matters Most

JOHN ENSOR

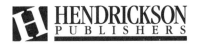

Pregnancy Crisis Intervention: What to Do and Say When It Matters Most

© 2019 John Ensor

Hendrickson Publishers Marketing, LLC
P. O. Box 3473
Peabody, Massachusetts 01961-3473
www.hendrickson.com

ISBN 978-1-68307-207-2

All rights reserved. No part of this book may be reproduced or transmitted in any form or by any means, electronic or mechanical, including photocopying, recording, or by any information storage and retrieval system, without permission in writing from the publisher.

All Scripture quotations are taken from the Holy Bible, English Standard Version (ESV®), copyright © 2001, by Crossway, a publishing ministry of Good News Publishers. Used by permission. All rights reserved.

Printed in the United States of America

First Printing—January 2019

Library of Congress Cataloging-in-Publication Data

A catalog record for this title is available from the Library of Congress
Hendrickson Publishers Marketing, LLC ISBN 978-1-68307-207-2

CONTENTS

Introduction: The Need for Wise Engagement

"If I don't get an abortion, I'm going to..."

*"My heart throbs; my strength fails me,
and the light of my eyes—it also has gone from me."*

—Psalm 38:10

The phone rang. The caller's voice quivered as she told me she was sixteen years old. Her emotions were so intense that she spoke haltingly. *"If I don't get . . . an abortion . . . I'm going to kill myself."* Before I could respond, she revealed her full anguish. *"But I know after my abortion, I won't be able to . . . I will need to kill myself."*

This teenager is experiencing crisis—a pregnancy-related crisis. Based on abortion rates worldwide, it is probable that more people around the world experience crisis from unexpected pregnancy than any other event.[1] The Guttmacher Institute Fact Sheet "Global Incidence and Trends,"[2] based on the Lancet Research, reports the following:

- During 2010–14, an estimated 56 million induced abortions occurred each year worldwide. This number represents an increase from 50 million annually during 1990–94, mainly because of population growth.

- The global annual rate of abortion, estimated at 35 abortions per 1,000 women of childbearing age (i.e., those fifteen to forty-four years old) in 2010–14, has declined slightly, from forty per 1,000 in 1990–94.

- Globally, 25 percent of pregnancies ended in abortion in 2010–14. In developed countries, the proportion declined from 39 percent to 28 percent between 1990–94 and 2010–14, whereas it increased from 21 percent to 24 percent in developing countries.

Yet, because pregnancy is common and normal and abortion is legal and accessible in most places, many will discount the reality of pregnancy crisis. *"If you want a baby, give birth. If you don't want a baby, get an abortion. Where's the crisis?"*

My caller revealed what many women experience—both options create deep and profound internal crisis. In acute panic and with distorted perspective, as teenagers are inclined to have, she revealed how her pregnancy was simply unbearable. Her pregnancy felt like death—the end of her life. True, her pregnancy was not a fatal disease, but it did present a mortal threat to her life *as she had projected it.* Getting an abortion was, in her mind, a life-saving necessity.

At the same moment, she expected that abortion, while resolving one crisis, would create another. Her contemplation of suicide subsequent to her abortion revealed a self-awareness that there was another stakeholder involved—her unborn child. Aborting her unborn presented itself as something wholly contrary to her self-image and pride in being a caring person. She anticipated not being able to live with the subsequent guilt and grief.

In short, my caller displayed the classic elements used within the professional field of crisis and trauma counseling (also known as CISM—critical incident stress management) that identify or define *crisis*. She also presented several specific elements associated with *pregnancy*-related crisis. In chapter 2, we will clarify the meaning of crisis and look at the specific indicators commonly presented in a pregnancy-related crisis.

Listening to the depth and extremity of my caller's desperation, I admit, created a momentary crisis in *me*. *"What if I say the wrong thing? What is the right thing to say at this critical moment? What if I lose her and she hangs up and then kills herself?"*

My first instinct was flight. I thought, *"I don't want to be the one she's talking to now."* I felt uncomfortable about learning more. *"If I don't know about such despair, then I won't feel the way I do right now."* But I knew that *"without my intervention right now, something fatal may happen. She needs me."*

Clearly, I was experiencing stress. I am a mature person with life experience and general counseling skills. Like *most* people working in the field of crisis intervention counseling, however, I was not a licensed, professionally trained expert in crisis intervention. But two who are, Burl E. Gilliland and Richard K. James, write:

> Contrary to the popular misconception that paid veteran crisis workers descend on a large-scale disaster like smoke-jumpers into a forest fire, most crisis intervention in the United States is done by volunteers. . . . Volunteerism is often the key to getting the fledgling crisis agency rolling. The use of trained volunteers as crisis workers has been a recognized component of many crisis centers and agencies for years.[3]

I was the one she reached out to. I was the one listening to her despair. I needed to understand my own role and stay calm if I was going to help her.

Crisis intervention trainer George S. Everly Jr. explains the need: *"Both* mental health clinicians and peer support personnel may perform crisis intervention and CISM services . . . but specialized training is essential for both groups."[4] The task requires the insights of crisis management and mental health professionals. Meeting the need requires volunteers and staff who serve as peer counselors.

In this book, we will use the term "peer counselor" or simply "counselor" to refer to those doing pregnancy crisis intervention (PCI). Within the field of pregnancy intervention services, various terms are used to define the person doing the intervention: peer counselor, client advocate, pregnancy consultant, and so on. Because "counselor" can imply a licensed professional, many pregnancy help organizations (PHOs) prefer the term "advocate" or "consultant." However, it is *accepted* practice within the field of crisis counseling for people to receive specialized, in-house training, and thereafter be referred to as "counselors." This is common in drug/alcohol addiction, divorce recovery, military reentry, and so on. Following this practice, a *counselor* implies *only* that the person has been trained and authorized by the PHO to serve women and couples in crisis.

Understanding who we are as peer counselors in the context of pregnancy crisis intervention is the focus of chapter 3.

My caller was full of fear. My immediate response was to assure her that she had called the right place and that I was going to help her. My goal in saying this was to lower her fear just a tick. Creating an atmosphere of calm is prerequisite to clearer thinking. Clearer thinking is the runway for wise decision-making and, hopefully, a life-affirming resolution. Understanding these goals and guiding the person's thinking and decision-making with emotional awareness and accurate information is the focus of chapter 4.

Abortion is fraught with emotion and moral upheaval. In chapter 5, we outline the principle of informed consent and present the legal and medical justification for talking about abortion with honesty and accuracy, in spite of the discomfort that may attend it.

Pregnancy crisis intervention unfolds like a story. There is a beginning: where people meet and the tone is set, and the characters, occasions, and choices leading to the crisis are told. There is a middle: where, having listened to her plight and taken note of the elements of deception, bad choices, missing information, and false expectations that are part of her story, you begin to speak. There are usually one or two "aha" moments, where a streak of light breaks in on a pathway that seemed nonexistent before. As the session reaches a conclusion, a bonding relationship is forged, and you take the first steps on that new pathway together. In chapter 6, we discuss the phases of crisis intervention from assessment to resolution.

Finally, in chapter 7 we explore the intervention skills that are vital to pregnancy crisis intervention—skills that can be developed and improved with intentional effort.

To help you grasp the central lessons of pregnancy crisis intervention, I've asked for illustrations, further insights, or additional, even differing, perspectives from leaders working in pregnancy help organizations. These "voices from the field" come from those with many years of experience doing pregnancy crisis intervention.

My caller was young. Her perspective was clouded. But she was not crazy. She saw herself as a loving person who would never intentionally hurt another human being, especially a child—especially her own child. Her extreme language was her way of expressing what lies at the heart of a pregnancy-related crisis: the humanity of the unborn.

If the unborn is not human, then destroying it does not need to be justified by critical circumstances any more than you need critical circumstances to justify cutting your hair. If the unborn is human, however, then there are no circumstances—no matter how painful—that justify killing the unborn child, any more than those same circumstances would justify killing a two-year-old. This is the ethical/moral crisis at the heart of the matter.

Upholding the humanity of the unborn while affirming the woman in crisis and eventually finding a life-affirming solution for both is the central challenge of pregnancy crisis intervention. It's a profoundly challenging but ultimately rewarding work for all involved. This book is written to help you be good at it—to know with confidence what to do and say when it matters most.

Starting Points in What to Do and Say When It Matters Most

"All you need is love, love. Love is all you need."

—John Lennon

For the whole law is fulfilled in one word:
"You shall love your neighbor as yourself."

—Galatians 5:14

A pregnancy related crisis may present itself to you in the form of a daughter, a sister, a schoolmate, a close friend, or a co-worker. You are not a licensed professional counselor. But you are the one she turned to for counsel.

For most readers of this book, that crisis will present itself as someone seeking services from a pregnancy help organization (PHO). You have come to your local PHO and are in training to work regularly with women and couples experiencing pregnancy-related crisis.

Beginners often experience trepidation in entering into the crisis of others. It isn't, however, competence you lack. It's confidence. You don't realize that while, of course, you need to learn more and improve your skills to make you more effective, you already have everything you need right now to do an adequate job of pregnancy crisis intervention. Counseling is properly understood to be "a conversation where one party with questions, problems, and trouble seeks assistance from someone they believe has answers, solutions, and help."[1] Lots of people, then, are good counselors.

Remember, there is no such thing as a professional mother or auntie. You can't get a masters degree in friendship. You don't need to be licensed as a good neighbor in order to be one. On any given day, around the world, there are moms, aunties, BFF's, and good neighbors who are approached by someone in a pregnancy crisis and who prove to be good counselors. They have not read this book, but they will do and say the right things when it matters most.

Why is that possible? Because they love the person in crisis, and love is the actual life-saving power in pregnancy crisis intervention.

When someone is in crisis, they are in a state of emotional disequilibrium. They are in inner turmoil. In pregnancy related crises, the dominant emotion that has metastasized out of control is *fear*. As the fear grows, it then paralyzes normative patterns of thinking and decision-making. Lower the fear and normative processes of coping and problem-solving reemerge. As already noted, the reason untrained people can figure out what to do and say when approached by someone in a crisis pregnancy is because they love the person in crisis. This love guides their words and actions and diminishes fear. For example, love naturally teaches you to listen. Listening signals empathy. For the person in crisis, just finding someone who cares enough to listen relieves fear and stress. To them, you are like the proverbial shelter in the raging storm. Although nothing in their circumstances has changed, they begin to relax emotionally. They share their broken heart with you, and then open their heart to your counsel.

It's your love for the woman in crisis that intuitively guides you to slow things down and make sure she obtains the pregnancy-related information necessary to make an informed decision. It's love that prompts you to ask hard questions, even ones she may not be eager to consider. Love is gritty that way. As your conversation ends, it's love that prompts you to say, "I will help you. We'll get through this together."

If you can love, then you can do pregnancy crisis intervention. Our point is not that love *alone* is all you need for effective crisis counseling, but it is all you need *to get started.* Good training is still necessary, because people do and say much that is insensitive to those in crisis, and people in crisis have specific needs. Love alone does not provide information, but it does provide motivation. Love, then, is the foundation for effective crisis intervention and a guiding power in applying all that you study and learn in pregnancy crisis intervention.

Using this as our foundation, we offer three further starting points for the beginner:

1. One rule
2. One illustration
3. One sentence

These will reduce the complex dynamics and the counseling approaches explored in this book down to easily remembered, simple, and recognizable starting points.

The One Rule

The Golden Rule is golden precisely because it has universal value and is always effective: "So whatever you wish that others would do to you, do also for them" (Matthew 7:12). Not only is this a rule for living in general, but it works especially well as a guide for pregnancy crisis intervention.

Pregnancy crisis intervention begins with a sympathizing imagination. If you can imagine yourself as the woman or couple telling you their story, and you feel what they feel, then you will likely say and do the right things in general. Yes, of course this book aims to provide you with in-depth understanding and improved skills relative to pregnancy intervention. But it's just as true to say that this book aims to help you follow the Golden Rule with greater insight and effectiveness. Trust the rule. It's golden.

Love Your Neighbor as Yourself
"My Start"

When I started, I knew only two things, and that was after going through a crisis pregnancy with my fifteen-year-old. One, I knew women in crisis needed a safe, loving place to talk. I've got plenty of love and compassion for young women in crisis and knew that I could give them the time and space they needed. Two, I knew God wanted me to help others through troubled waters. I had no expertise, but that was my heart.

I started out as a calm listener who was there to ask questions, and with each answer, to help them to find their way out of the woods. Now I've got seventeen years of experience. So let me assure you, if you listen to their hearts, they will hear yours. That's a good start.

—Vikki Parker, Option Pregnancy Center

The One Illustration

The paradigm illustration for all crisis intervention is the story of the Good Samaritan (Luke 10:25–37):

And behold, a lawyer stood up to put him to the test, saying, "Teacher, what shall I do to inherit eternal life?" He said to him, "What is written in the Law? How do you read it?" And he answered, "You shall love the Lord your God with all your heart and with all your soul and with all your strength and with all your mind, and your neighbor as yourself." And he said to him, "You have answered correctly; do this, and you will live."

But he, desiring to justify himself, said to Jesus, "And who is my neighbor?" Jesus replied, "A man was going down from Jerusalem to Jericho, and he fell among robbers, who stripped him and beat him and departed, leaving him half dead. Now by chance a priest was going down that road, and when he saw him he passed by on the other side. So likewise a Levite, when he came to the place and saw him, passed by on the other side. But a Samaritan, as he journeyed, came to where he was, and when he saw him, he had compassion. He went to him and bound up his wounds, pouring on oil and wine. Then he set him on his own animal and brought him to an inn and took care of him. And the next day he took out two denarii and gave them to the innkeeper, saying, 'Take care of him, and whatever more you spend, I will repay you when I come back.' Which of these three, do you think, proved to be a neighbor to the man who fell among the robbers?" He said, "The one who showed him mercy." And Jesus said to him, "You go, and do likewise."

This story, like the Golden Rule, is recognized in the culture at large and is a quick reference point to all works of emergency intervention. People often say, "We didn't know what we were going to do, but then this Good Samaritan showed up."

A Good Samaritan is one who is motivated and guided by compassion. Compassion means "to suffer with." Compassion is the ability to imagine the needs of others as if they were your own. It is empathy converted into intervention. You have compassion when you can make the problems of others your problems and, in return, convert your strength and resources into the temporary strength and resources they need. We say temporary, because crisis intervention is short-term help that ends when a person reestablishes their normal coping/problem-solving abilities.

The parable of the Good Samaritan serves as a good paradigm for crisis intervention, because the context for the story told is crisis—a matter of life and death. A man was left to die and will die without direct intervention. The moral urgency of preventing an innocent human being from unjustly being killed guides the Samaritan's direct acts of intervention.

The Samaritan figures out what to do and does it with love as his guide. This love prompts one thing, then another, and so on, until the man's life is rescued. Another way to say this is that the Samaritan freely does for the dying man what he imagines wishing someone would do for him if he were beaten, robbed, and left to die.

Likewise, crisis intervention involves drawing near to the person in crisis, doing some immediate triage, and then personally helping them stabilize and develop a plan forward. What is unique to pregnancy crisis intervention is the need to see that two people are at risk: the mother and her unborn child.

Dr. Bernard Nathanson, a former abortion advocate and practitioner, changed his approach to pregnancy crisis when, through ultrasound, he saw two people involved in the crisis:

> From then on we could see this person in the womb from the very beginning—and study and measure it and weigh it and take care of it and treat it and diagnose it and do all kinds of things. It became, in essence, a second patient. Now a patient is a person. So basically, I was dealing then with two people, instead of just one carrying some lump of meat around. That's what started me doubting the ethical acceptability of abortion on requests.[2]

Our specialized goal in pregnancy crisis intervention is to provide the practical help and emotional support necessary for both mother and child to survive the crisis and live well.

The One Sentence

When you first engage in PCI, you will be tempted to keep before you everything you learn in this book. Don't do that. Instead, remember this one-sentence summary: *Speak the truth in love.* Focus on these five words and you will recall the parts of this book that you need when you need them.

"Speak the truth in love" is a perfectly balanced starting point for PCI. Truth without love is like a bright light shone into your eyes on a dark night. It reflexively causes you to turn away (and get angry at the person pointing it). Truth *with* love is like a flashlight pointed onto the dark, winding, jagged path before you. It invites looking to see the sure-footed next step and reveals missteps to avoid.

Love without truth is like the proverbial frog in the water: warm and comfortable but blind to the deadly danger of the hot stove. In the end, love without truth is more likely about being loved rather than loving. Love without truth is often cowardly silence or the fear of rejection, masked as support.

The work of PCI is predicated on truth and love working together. The truth is the bioethical, scientific truth: the humanity of the unborn. The law of love is the principal law for all human relationships: Love your neighbor as yourself. Talk to anyone who works in any of the four thousand-plus PHOs worldwide, and you will discover that they have no special secrets other than this: They love those in crisis and speak the truth in love to them.

"Ready, Fire, Aim!"

A final word to beginners: Do not underestimate the power of "ready, fire, aim!"

Yes, the following chapters will make you a better counselor. But for beginners, the real obstacle is a lack of confidence due to a lack of experience. Only by engaging a frightened woman in a pregnancy-related crisis will you eventually become both confident and competent. You may think you need to learn more before you can do more. I suggest, however, that you eagerly do your best and you will learn more as you go.

Nobody gets to do PCI work with a guarantee of a good and satisfying outcome all the time. This is true of emergency relief workers, trauma specialists, and crisis counselors in every field. We are dealing with extraordinary circumstances, deep trauma, and broken people. Training is vital to the work, but experience is the curing process of true knowledge. "Ready, fire, aim" is the best way to get to "ready, aim, fire!"

2

Understanding Crisis and the Woman in a Pregnancy-Related Crisis

"I told Dad I wouldn't have the abortion, but he said I was going to have it anyway—that it was for my own good."

—Janet

"I am weary with moaning;
every night I flood my bed with tears;
I drench my couch with my weeping."

—Psalm 6:6

There are several indicators common to all human crises. Then there are particular ways women in a pregnancy-related crisis present themselves. Pregnancy crisis intervention begins with understanding crises in general and women in pregnancy crisis in particular.

Society's attempt to understand human crises and construct models of intervention is a recent development within the broader field of psychology and counseling. In 1944, Gerald Caplan and Erich Lindemann were the first to analyze the dynamics of human crisis and publish a model of intervention.

Lisa Jackson-Cherry and Bradley Erford summarize this pioneering effort:

> Their work began after the tragic Cocoanut Grove Nightclub fire in Boston, in which so many people died in Boston in 1942. . . . Based on his interviews with those who survived the fire as well as survivors of the deceased, Lindemann outlined a number of common clinical features, including somatic distress, feelings of guilt, hostility, disorganization, behavioral changes, and preoccupation with images of the deceased. Lindemann referred to these symptoms as "acute grief," which was not a psychiatric diagnosis but was a call for intervention nonetheless.[1]

Since that time, the field of crisis assessment and management has developed apace. The textbook *Crisis Assessment, Intervention, and Prevention* reflects this development and application. The first section describes current theories and approaches to crisis intervention and outlines the formative dynamics of crisis as a human experience.

The second section, accounting for two-thirds of the textbook, gets specific. It dedicates a chapter to understanding and treating each of the following crises: substance abuse, intimate partner violence, sexual assault, child sexual assault, emergency response in the workplace, emergency response in schools, military deployment and reentry issues, and death notification.

There is no chapter on pregnancy crisis intervention and management.[2] The same is true for the standard textbook *Crisis Intervention Strategies*, now in its eighth edition.[3] It begins with the theory of crisis intervention and related approaches, and it ends with specific applications for situations including sexual assault, partner violence, bereavement and grief, disaster response, and more. They do not, however, address the crisis induced by an unplanned pregnancy. Why is that?

For over forty-five years now, PHOs have been working on pregnancy-related crisis and intervention, longer in fact than attention has been given to some of the crisis areas listed above.[4] As of this writing, there are 2,829 pregnancy help organizations in the United States alone.[5] Outside the States—in South America, Canada, Africa, Europe, and Asia—there are an additional 2,653 PHOs. These emerged out of a grassroots movement of volunteers responding to local need. They gained experience in meeting those needs, and they shared their experiences with new volunteers. Over time, manuals, conferences, and training organizations developed.

This development is in keeping with the whole history of crisis intervention as a profession. As Gilliland and James write,

> To really understand the evolution of crisis intervention, though, is to understand that several social movements have been critical to its development, and these did not start fully formed as "crisis intervention" groups by any means. Three of the major movements that helped shaped crisis intervention into an emerging specialty were Alcoholics Anonymous (AA), Vietnam veterans, and the women's movement of the 1970s. Although their commissioned intentions and objectives had little to do with the advancement of crisis intervention as a clinical specialty.[6]

As a grassroots movement grows, it does develop an expertise and becomes recognized in the field of crisis intervention. A recent example, in parallel to the pregnancy help movement, is Mothers Against Drunk Driving. It started out as volunteers deciding to address the crisis of drunk driving since no one else did. It eventually produced sufficient societal attention to change policy and law and created a new category for crisis intervention.

Suicide prevention also started out as a volunteer hotline. Addiction intervention emerged from the grassroots of volunteers, many of whom had struggled with addiction themselves, forming groups under the name of Alcoholics Anonymous. Postwar PTSD treatment started in storefronts, run by volunteers—again, many of whom had struggled with it themselves. In other words, one explanation for why PCI has not yet been formally recognized within the profession is one of developmental maturity as a movement.

But just as likely an explanation for why pregnancy crisis intervention has not yet been recognized professionally may be that the politics of abortion itself make it difficult to recognize pregnancy-related crisis. It requires separating the political from the professional. Individually that may happen, but universities, professional accreditation organizations, and research journals are now viewpoint-based.

The viewpoint adopted by these institutions is that the trauma historically related to pregnancy has been addressed and solved politically, by making contraception and abortion legal and available. To the extent that pregnancy crisis remains a problem, the political solution of more contraception and improved abortion services are considered the solution. For example, the fact sheet on "Induced Abortion Worldwide," published by the Guttmacher Institute, concludes, "In many settings, young women are disadvantaged with respect to their ability to access contraception and safe abortion."[7] What is lacking in this perspective is a serious examination of the psychology of pregnancy-related crisis itself.

When we examine pregnancy crisis, we find that most women seeking an abortion self-identify as people who do not believe in abortion and do not want one. In one study,

> Fully 64 percent of the aborted women surveyed described themselves as "forced" into abortion because of their particular circumstances at the time. Most of these women also indicated that during the time between discovering they were pregnant and having the abortion there was such a high level of emotional trauma that they were unable to thoughtfully and cautiously consider their

alternatives. Abortion was simply the most obvious and fastest way to escape from their dilemmas. Over 84 percent state that they would have kept their babies under better circumstances.[8]

The woman in a pregnancy crisis will typically express her intentions with the voice of surrender: "I don't believe in abortion, but I have no choice." As Frederica Mathewes-Green put it, "No one wants an abortion as she wants an ice cream cone or a Porsche. She wants an abortion as an animal, caught in a trap, wants to gnaw off its own leg."[9]

What about those who have no moral reservations about either contraceptive use or elective abortion? Contraception promotes sexual activity under the promise of protection from pregnancy, and abortion access is the promised failsafe. As shown by the Alan Guttmacher Institute—the research arm of Planned Parenthood that specializes in contraception and abortion—54 percent of women coming for *abortion* were using *contraception* at the time of pregnancy.[10]

For many, however, abortion appears as the perfect failsafe, *right up to the point at which they find themselves pregnant* or find their partner pregnant. Then, no matter what one's perspective on elective abortion, actual pregnancy changes things. The innate desire to provide and protect clashes with one's immediate self-interest, and the inner conflict begins. These complex emotions and conflicting inner values are further intensified by a woman's difficult personal circumstances. These difficulties are usually related to the intense anxiety of being unmarried and unsure of the stability of the relationship. Finally, they are multiplied by the conflicting feelings and thoughts of her partner, parents, or friends. The result is an intense pregnancy-related crisis, no matter what one believes politically about elective abortion.

Perhaps the strongest indicator that pregnancy crisis is common and complex apart from one's beliefs about elective abortion is found in listening to women who suffered sexual assault and subsequent pregnancy. This is the most traumatizing context for pregnancy. Abortion researcher David Reardon writes,

> Typically, people on both sides of the abortion debate accept the premise that most women who become pregnant through sexual assault want abortions. From this "fact," it naturally follows that the reason women want abortions in these cases is because it will help them to put the assault behind them, recover more quickly, and avoid the additional trauma of giving birth to a "rapist's child."[11]

Yet, surprisingly, studies show that 75 percent of women who are pregnant as a result of rape resolve to carry to term.[12] Why is that? It's important to let women tell their own stories and for us to simply listen.[13] But the short answer is that the experience of pregnancy is not the politics of abortion.

Professionals in crisis intervention and assessment should appreciate the trauma that women experience from an unexpected pregnancy and respond with the dignity, respect, and professionalism they bring to other areas of human crisis.

Understanding Human Crisis in General

In the field of crisis management, a crisis refers to the emotional upheaval people experience following an acute precipitating event that is not alleviated by customary coping resources. Gerald Caplan provides the following description:

> People are in a state of crisis when they face an obstacle to important life goals—an obstacle that is, for a time, insurmountable by the use of customary methods of problem-solving. A period of disorganization ensues, a period of upset, during which many abortive attempts at solution [*sic*] are made.[14]

Douglas A. Puryear, in his book *Helping People in Crisis,* further develops our recognition of crisis.[15] A state of crisis is characterized by:

1. Symptoms of stress
    The person in crisis is experiencing both psychological and physiological stress in ways that can include headaches, depression, anxiety, bleeding ulcers, etc.

2. An attitude of panic or defeat
    A person who has tried every way he can to solve a problem and has failed feels overwhelmed, inadequate, and helpless. He will tend to be either agitated, with unproductive behavior . . . or he will tend to be apathetic (retreating into bed or into a drunken stupor).

3. A focus on relief
    In this state a person is primarily interested in relief of the pain of stress—the headache, the depression. . . . There is little gathering or noticing of new facts or new ideas, and little organized effort at problem-solving. Relief will generally be sought by discharge behavior, withdrawal behavior, or turning to others for rescue.

4. A time of lowered efficiency
    In this state a person may continue to function normally, but his efficiency is markedly lower, and those problem-solving efforts that persist are inefficient.

5. A limited duration
    People cannot exist in this state for long—it is unbearable. It will end and a state of equilibrium be regained within a maximum of six weeks.

These indications are common to people in an active state of crisis, no matter what the antecedent may be (tornado, sexual assault, terrorist attack, and so on). Anyone with even minimal experience in pregnancy crisis intervention will recognize that these indications also accurately describe the way women or couples struggling with an unexpected pregnancy present themselves.

Understanding the Woman in Pregnancy Crisis

Effective pregnancy crisis intervention begins with understanding how these general indications of human crisis present themselves, particularly in women experiencing a pregnancy-related crisis.

Though crisis is idiosyncratic—and each woman brings her own cognitive, emotional, and behavioral reactions to her crisis experience—patterns emerge. As you listen, you will see her present her crisis in seven characteristic ways.

VOICES FROM THE FIELD

Understanding the Woman
"The Dignity of Motherhood"

Young mothers in pregnancy crisis are typically in unhealthy situations, making unhealthy choices out of their insecurity or sense of failure. No one has ever assured them of the quiet beauty and dignity of changing diapers, rocking a child with a fever, or playing peek-a-boo. Last year in Maine, almost 52 percent of abortions were to moms who had at least one prior birth. These moms lacked confidence in being mothers. They are often blind to the high calling of motherhood itself.

Jessica was a single mom who came to our PHO intending abortion. I asked her why she thought that was her best option. She explained that in her previous pregnancy, the doctor immediately referred her for an abortion. The doctor made her feel like: "No way can you handle this. Abortion is your only option." Jessica told me, "I defied him!" Now here she was several years later with a toddler. Her thinking was: "I beat the odds once. But certainly, I can't do it twice!" This, of course, is false and I addressed it. At our second visit, Jessica sheepishly said, "After our first visit, I realized I'm a pretty good mom! Maybe I can parent a second child." I looked her square in the eye and said, "Of course you can." The tears that welled up in her eyes spoke volumes. She participated in our parenting education and support program to learn all she could to be the best mom she could be.

—Tina Williams, Alpha Pregnancy Resource Center

1. She is fearful.

From the earliest suggested indication of pregnancy, she experiences fear. This fear may begin right after intercourse, simply because of knowing what might happen. As indications of pregnancy appear (late period, swollen breasts, etc.), the fear increases. By the time a simple urine pregnancy test is taken, panic is setting in.

The fear is unremitting. She thinks of the significant people in her life and pictures their response to her pregnancy. She considers how having a baby will shatter her current plans for school or her career. As she thinks of her options, *each one* adds to her fear.

Her fear is organic—unlike the safe, self-induced fear she may experience watching a horror film. In that context, she is still in control. She can close her eyes and make it go away. Pregnancy crisis is a palpable fear precisely because of this loss of control. She thinks, "This cannot be happening to me." But it is.

Voices from the Field

She Is Fearful

"Paralyzing Fear"

I've had callers who made several attempts to call but hung up before I could answer. This is how debilitating fear can be. The young woman can be afraid even to voice her desperation and ask for help, because doing so confirms a truth she's been denying to this moment: "I'm pregnant."

—Jeanne Pernia, PassionLife

2. She is under pressure.

The woman in pregnancy crisis will express feeling tremendous pressure. This pressure is both internal and external in origin.

Internally, pregnancy may represent a failure of her moral or religious values. These women or couples may hold to a clear code of sexual ethics, but they have not found the strength and maturity required to live according to this code. The guilt is acute. The shame of exposure is also acute. Typically, the first response to moral failure is a resolve to "never do that again." Soon a pattern emerges: sexual activity followed by guilt and shame, followed by moral resolution that soon fails. Over time, a secret life or lifestyle emerges. Pregnancy threatens to reveal all.

For the nonreligious, or secularist, sexual behavior is governed primarily by only one moral absolute: sex must be consensual. But sociologically, the human spirit resists this reduction. Sex continues to mean something for most people beyond the consensual activity itself. Sex changes things. It realigns the relationship. It sets up new expectations. Sex resulting in pregnancy places those expectations under extreme pressure. It is normal for women to want their partners to support them.

Even when the pressure appears to come externally—say, from parents—the actual pressure may be internal. For example, it is not unusual for an eighteen-year-old to express confidence that her parents are loving and supportive and would help her carry to term. Still, she doesn't want to disappoint them or embarrass them by her sexual choices and the shame of an out-of-wedlock birth.

Externally, the pressure typically comes from her partner, family, and friends. According to Frederica Mathewes-Green, who surveyed reasons women give for having an abortion, the highest percentage (38.2 percent) reported that they resorted to abortion in response to pressure from a husband or a boyfriend.[16] In another survey, David Reardon concludes, "The opinions and pressures of others play a major role in the final decision of most aborting women. . . . *Nearly 55% of the respondents felt they had been very much 'forced' to abort by others.*" He also notes that 51 percent of the time, this other person was a husband or boyfriend.[17]

The following account shows how extensive this external pressure can be. Notice that nothing in this woman's decision was about freedom or privacy, power, or rights. It was about feeling under pressure.

> My family would not support my decision to keep the baby. My boyfriend said he would give me no emotional or financial help whatsoever. All the people that mattered told me to abort. When I said I didn't want to, they started listing reasons why I should. That it would have detrimental effects on my career, and my health, and that I would have no social life and no future with men. . . . I'm so angry at myself for giving in to the pressure of others.[18]

We can speak then of an individual in crisis. "But as crises unfold, they rarely remain confined to one person. They ripple out and affect numerous other people. . . . For most individuals the first ripple effect of a crisis will be with the family system."[19] In PCI this is almost always true. The father of the baby—as well as parents, siblings, and friends—are all responding to the pregnancy and are directly affecting the woman in pregnancy distress. Therefore, while our focus is on her in the counseling context, our intervention must address her system of support (or lack of support).

VOICES FROM THE FIELD

Under Pressure
"Some Men Are the Solution"

While it is true that most women seek abortions to please a man—some studies show this to be over 50 percent—that still leaves a large percentage of men who want to be good men and good fathers. Two men come to mind. One showed up with his mother, seeking help. His girlfriend intended abortion, but he wanted to respect life and take responsibility. Another came in with his girlfriend, and they were divided over what to do. Both men were in crisis to protect their unborn child. They sought our guidance in how to talk about the issues. Both men spoke up and showed genuine support and care for their girlfriends. Both women eventually gave birth and let these fathers raise their babies.

It's tempting to treat men and fathers like the enemy. They're not. In pregnancy crisis intervention work, we meet lots of good men who have a passion to be great fathers.

—Melinda Gardner, Apple Pregnancy Care Center

3. She sees her pregnancy as life-threatening.

The woman in pregnancy crisis often sees her pregnancy as a life versus life situation. Apart from rare medical conditions, this is not true. But it feels true.

It is true in this sense: her pregnancy does threaten her life *as she has projected it.* Pregnancy, no matter what the outcome (parenting, abortion, or adoption) is unavoidably a life-changing experience.

All crises—whether it be the death of a friend, sexual assault, or a house-destroying fire—arise from an actual life-changing experience. It's happened and it can't be undone, ever. The first response, however, is to cry "No! This cannot be happening to me." It does represent the end of one's life as currently planned and experienced day by day. It remains a crisis until such time that people accept the new norm and adjust. In other words, crisis forces growth.

When people refuse to adjust and grow in response to traumatic events, it changes them nonetheless, just in unhealthy ways. Charles Dickens explored this dynamic in his novel *Great Expectations*. The character of Miss Havisham refused to adjust in any way to the loss of her fiancé on her wedding day, refusing to ever remove her wedding dress. But as the story shows, change is a constant. The only question is whether we embrace it in healthy or unhealthy ways.

You are talking to someone who doesn't want her life to change and has not yet accepted that the precipitating experience of her crisis, the pregnancy, has forever changed her life already. In some cases, she may be ready to accept the change but is under severe pressure from others who don't want their lives changed by her pregnancy. Either way, pregnancy in this context feels like a death sentence. From this perspective, abortion then is a justifiable life-saving solution. The abortion doctor is the true savior.

You may never have thought about abortion in such terms. You may, in fact, think very differently. If your context is serving in a PHO, then you probably see abortion as the intentional killing of an innocent human being. She may even agree to a large extent. You will often hear women in pregnancy distress say, "I know it's wrong, but I have no choice." What she means by this is, "I know abortion kills a baby, but I have the right to save my own life."

Effective pregnancy intervention requires understanding this psychological perspective. You are thinking that if a woman knows abortion is wrong, then she should not make that choice, no matter the difficulty of her circumstances. True enough. But *at this point,* she's not seeing things that clearly. She sees it much more as a life versus life scenario. To her at that moment, abortion is a life-saving solution.

Brianna Cain is one of six women interviewed for an online article titled "Abortion: The Most Important Decision of Her Life." Notice how she sees her abortion as a life-saving action:

> "There was something inside of me that I didn't want and that was in conflict with how I wanted my life to be," she said. . . . "It allowed me to continue my life," she said of having two abortions.[20]

Celina Perez writes her account in *Cosmopolitan* magazine:

> Having an abortion saved my life then, and it made my life now. Something I hear a lot is, "What about adoption?" How was I supposed to carry a kid for nine months when I worked two jobs that are physically demanding? People don't think about what it really means to make these choices when it isn't them. I wouldn't be the person I am—a successful, happy person—if I had to have that baby. I would be somebody stuck in poverty with few options to dig out of it. I didn't become a heart surgeon or win a Nobel Prize. I just became an independent person who was able to find happiness. The opportunity to do that is the least anyone deserves.[21]

On January 22, 2016, the anniversary of the *Roe v. Wade* decision, Janice MacAvoy submitted a Friend-of-the-Court brief asking the Supreme Court to strike down a Texas law aimed at closing abortion clinics in the state: "To the world, I am an attorney who had an abortion, and, to myself, I am an attorney because I had an abortion."[22]

One final example. In an interview with TV personality Tavis Smiley, Gloria Steinem, the feminist icon and abortion rights activist, recalled her own abortion as a young woman: "It gave me my life. I mean, I wouldn't have been able to live my life otherwise."[23]

In all four of these examples, abortion is seen as a life-preserving action in the sense that it liberated these women to pursue their personal life goals.

4. She seeks quick relief.

People can live with crisis for only so long. Then they will take action to end it—some action, any action, even if that means ending their own lives. One crisis intervention specialist, Dr. H. Norman Wright, suggests that on average, people will resolve their crisis one way or another "within a period of six weeks."[24] This is also true for those in crisis over an unexpected pregnancy.

For those in a pregnancy-related crisis, the combination of fear, inner and external pressure, and a sense of one's life spinning out of control creates an urgency to act. Ending the crisis and regaining control *as soon as possible* is integral to the experience of pregnancy distress.

The first question you are likely to hear on the phone when speaking to a woman in pregnancy crisis is "How much are your abortions?" It will not be "What are the procedures for an eight-week surgical abortion, and what are the risks associated with it?" The sense of urgency precludes gathering information, filtering options, understanding risks and outcomes, looking at alternative treatments—all of the due diligence questions she would ask, as people generally do, when considering any other kind of surgical procedure. Her demeanor, if not the actual expression, says, "I don't care anymore. I just want this situation to end. I can't take it anymore." The cognitive dissonance has stolen her sleep. The anxiety has wrung her dry. She doesn't want to think. She wants to stop thinking and get her old life back as fast as possible.

Understand, then, why many women and couples perceive abortion as the best option: it is the quickest solution.

For this reason, a good portion of the after-abortion grief reported by women has to do with a failure to understand at the time just what abortion is and the immediate and long-term risks. They did not know because they did not ask. They did not ask because that would have slowed things down and they were in a hurry to end the crisis.

Unfortunately, those who profit in the decision have no incentive to raise questions or operate under the principle of informed consent. Things are minimized or avoided, and a conspiracy of silence is created.

5. She has two minds/hears two voices.

Another helpful way to understand the woman in pregnancy crisis is to appreciate the inner conflict she has regarding abortion itself. This is true no matter what she thinks politically about legal abortion.

A woman presenting herself in a pregnancy-related crisis will almost always reveal ambivalence. She will express two minds: "I don't want an abortion," and "I want an abortion." The most common expression of these competing desires is the often-heard statement, "I really don't want an abortion, but I have no choice."

She's of two minds because she is wrestling with two voices. One is saying, "Don't do it. Things will work out." The other is saying, "Do it. Get the abortion. It's okay."

One voice, the softer of the two, appeals to the natural instinct to protect human life. She may recognize it as the voice of conscience, or "the fear of God," or simply the heartfelt values that come from a self-image of being a caring person who would never hurt another. This voice speaks to her inner strength as a human being. "You can do it! You do have the strength to have this baby, then parent or place for adoption." "You can finish school without sacrificing your core beliefs and values." This voice speaks to moral law and the obedience that comes from faith. "Do not murder. Do the right thing. Trust God to provide."

The other voice is pragmatic and much louder. Sometimes this is literally true in the sense that they are the voices of her boyfriend, friends, or family. The loud voice is reacting to the immediate difficulties of having a baby. "You can't afford it." "You'll end up on welfare." You'll never finish school." "Your parents will kill you!" "I'm not ready to be a father." "You can't do it alone." This voice does not so much argue against conscience as shout over it.

In the field of counseling a clash of ideas or values is called cognitive dissonance. In this context, you will see it as a genuine inner battle of two desires. On one side, there is moral vision regarding human value and rights and a belief that God will provide or things will work out in the end. On the other side, there is a sense of the rightness of moral autonomy and self-determination where the ends justify the means. As feminist author Naomi Wolf writes, it's about "our bodies and our souls."[25]

VOICES FROM THE FIELD

She Feels Alone
"I Showed All the Signs"

In my own pregnancy crisis, I remember experiencing every one of these pregnancy-related markers: I was under great pressure, and I became so afraid. I wanted my baby, but no one in my life at that time said that it was okay. The pressure was so great that I psyched myself into believing that with all the crying I did, and not eating or sleeping correctly due to the stress, that "surely my baby would not be normal." This is how I prepared myself to do want I did not want to do. I thought, "I should abort, because surely my baby would not be able to survive everything I was enduring."

At the time, my mother was operating an abortion business and I worked there too. On a Sunday morning, I aborted my first child in our own abortion business. If just one person had said "Jeannie, you're strong. You can have your baby!" things would have been different.

What a young woman often needs (even more than practical help) is someone who can stand by her when she says, in spite of her difficulties, "I want my baby." Roll up your sleeves then and say, "Okay, let's make it happen."

—Jeanne Pernia, PassionLife

6. She feels alone.

She may be encircled by siblings, friends, parents, and other advisors. Yet she feels alone. After all, she is the only one who will get on the table if she chooses abortion. If she has the baby, she fears her partner will leave her alone to raise the child. In some cases, she has been warned that this will happen. In other cases, she just fears that she does not have the support system needed to raise a child.

If she wants her baby, she may be the only one. In such cases, she faces ridicule and contempt, if not threats. Her boyfriend may tell her, "If you don't get an abortion, we're done. I'm out!" Parents may threaten to turn her out of the home or revoke college tuition payments, leaving her abandoned. The result is a profound alienation. As the psalmist cried, "Even my close friend in whom I trusted, who ate my bread, has lifted his heel against me" (Psalm 41:9).

In these situations, abortion is not so much a choice but a resignation. She's not seeking abortion as a self-actualizing power-encounter. She feels weak primarily because she feels alone.

7. She feels hopeless.

Pregnancy is an entirely natural occurrence. It's neither a disease nor a disability. It's not naturally a crisis. When occurring within a stable relationship during normal times (absent the duress of war or natural disaster, for example), getting pregnant is a hopeful development. It points to new life and to new possibilities and potentials.

But pregnancy within an unstable relationship, or outside the moral boundaries of one's sexual ethics, or under the duress of difficult economic circumstances, turns a naturally hopeful development into an utterly despairing situation.

The culminating effect of all the above descriptions is a feeling of hopelessness. The woman (or couple) simply cannot see how she can afford a baby at this point. She cannot see any possible way to finish school and also have a baby. She cannot see any support for what naturally is a two-parent task.

Understand, then, this is the woman who has come to see you. She feels hopeless and alone, conflicted and fearful. Her life appears over. Only drastic measures can rescue her—measures so drastic that she fears them too. Now she has come to you for help.

3

Understanding Who You Are in the Intervention Process

*"As long as it takes, no matter the challenges,
I find a way for mothers to make a choice
they, and their babies, can live with."*

—Jeanne Pernia, PassionLife

*"I was eyes to the blind and feet to the lame.
I was a father to the needy,
and I searched out the cause of him whom I did not know.
I broke the fangs of the unrighteous
and made him drop his prey from his teeth."*

—Job 29:15–17

Within minutes, the person who comes to talk to you about her crisis pregnancy is telling you personal, even intimate, details of her life. If the context for that discussion is inside a pregnancy help organization (PHO) or on the phone or hotline as a representative of the PHO, you are asking her invasive questions you would never ask under normal circumstances. For examples, you will need to ask about her recent sexual behavior, prior pregnancies and outcomes, the nature of her relationship with her partner, her deepest values, her religious beliefs, and most of all, why being pregnant at this time is so distressing.

Even as you focus on her and her story, you are filled with a high degree of self-awareness. You understand that you are playing a critical role in her life right now. What you say and do over the next thirty minutes to an hour truly does matter. That awareness can be intimidating. There are, however, concepts in self-understanding and principles of self-care that allow you to enter into the crises of others without creating your own internal crisis.

Understanding Who You Are in the Intervention Process

There are at least six ways to view yourself in the role of pregnancy crisis intervention. These concepts do not need to be memorized but simply realized and relied on, until your own experience in pregnancy intervention produces the confident and calm professional bearing you seek.

1. You are a loving person, so you use the love approach.

Love is the distillation of all Christian theology and ethics. As Christ taught,

> "You shall love the Lord your God with all your heart and with all your soul and with all your mind. This is the great and first commandment. And a second is like it: You shall love your neighbor as yourself. On these two commandments depend all the Law and the Prophets." (Matthew 22:37–40)

The love approach is all-pervasive and compelling. It applies not only to family and like-minded people but also to the stranger, the poor, the rude, the oppressive—even to one's enemies. Therefore, the approach you take to intervention is *always* the love approach.[1]

As you engage the woman in crisis, you don't know the outcome. You are mindful of your limits. You don't do magic, so you can't simply make the problem go away. Nor do you have abundant resources to quickly solve the challenges she faces. But you can have quiet confidence that the love of God you feel within you *is* the life-saving power you bring to her at this moment. Give it room to work. It will prompt you, so listen patiently. Convey a spirit of acceptance. Suspend judgment. Tell her you are sorry to see her in such a state.

Once she begins to tell her story, you will quickly observe that you're hearing a confession of sorts with painful, sometimes graphic, details. She may confess to lies she told and lies she believed. She may speak of manipulative plots to get what she wanted or manipulative tactics used to coerce her to do want she didn't want to do. She will tell you of some of the foolish (and sometimes illegal) choices she's made. You will quickly hear her assessment (perhaps accurate, perhaps not) of the relationship she has with the man involved; whether she perceives it as largely good and ongoing or mostly broken and about to end. You will also most likely hear her describe her parental or family dynamics—good and bad.

You are there to help her at this point going forward. You respond with politeness, respect, truthfulness, and patience. Why? Because that's what love does.

2. You bring a rescuer mentality to the crisis, so you make her a priority.

Everyone who works effectively in the field of crisis intervention brings a rescuer mentality to the job. As the psalmist says, "*Rescue* the weak and the needy" (Psalm 82:4; emphasis added). As a rule, however, thinking of yourself as a rescuer in the sense of being a savior is unwise, unhealthy, and untrue. I explain why later in this chapter.

Still, when the strong defend the weak, when the able help the disabled, when those who have help those in need, when voices are raised for the voiceless, such people are coming to the rescue of others. These are concrete actions of great value, and the plain word for these sorts of interventions is *rescue*.

Whether working as an emergency medical professional or bringing relief to a natural disaster area (flood, tornado, and so on), or helping a veteran struggling with the trauma of war or doing pregnancy crisis intervention, having a rescuer mentality concentrates the mind to triage the crisis and attend to the most critical and immediate needs. A rescuer mentality enables you to match the urgency of another's personal crisis with your own urgency of attention.

When the woman in pregnancy crisis sees that she is a priority concern for you, her fears will diminish a bit. Nothing in her circumstances has changed, but she sees that you take her fears seriously when others haven't or won't.

Having a rescuer mentality means you are sober minded and careful with your words. You say what you mean and mean what you say. If you make a promise, then you understand the absolute necessity of keeping it. If you don't, then you've added to her sense of crisis by becoming another person in her life who has failed her. So if you say, "I'll call you tomorrow," it's vital—no matter how busy you are—to call her the next day.

Having a rescuer mentality means you act with a calm urgency. This may sound like an oxymoron, like hot ice or dark light, but it's not. It's a controlled sense of urgency. Every rescuer needs this sense of calm urgency to function and sustain themselves in the work.

The rescuer mentality allows you to take temporary control in small but helpful ways when she is immobilized in fear and anxiety. It's called *directive* counseling to distinguish it from *facilitative* counseling. To grasp the difference, imagine you are on the phone with a young woman in pregnancy distress. Using a facilitative counseling approach, you ask her what time she can come in to the pregnancy help clinic for a pregnancy test and an ultrasound verification of pregnancy. But as I learned from experience, asking when she can come in can further increase her anxieties. All of a sudden, she's trying to recall her schedule from today till next year and she freezes up. A more directive approach is to ask, "Can you come in today at three o'clock?" That's a simple yes or no question and so much easier to process.

Also, "I want you to call me tomorrow" is stronger than "Will you call me tomorrow?" For those in crisis, the first statement is reassuring and signals to her that you care. It's not controlling or heavy-handed the way it might sound in the absence of a crisis.

Seeing yourself as a rescuer will help you communicate the priority that she is in your life and naturally speak in a more directive way when needed.

VOICES FROM THE FIELD

You Bring a Rescuer Mentality
"Focus on Them"

Talk about dropping all the distractions and concentrating on the woman in crisis! My first experience working at the PHO meant dealing with a crisis in the midst of a crisis. Our PHO office had opened only three days earlier when thieves broke in and stole our ultrasound machine. We had broken glass and blood on the floor. Reporters, police, and even CSI Miami investigators milled around, dusting for prints and asking questions. Our staff was crying. Then this couple walks in. "We need a pregnancy test and maybe an abortion," they said.

I forced myself to focus on their crisis alone. I walked them into a side room and sat down with them. I pushed all the noise and chaos out of my mind. We talked calmly about them and their crisis. Sure enough, that baby lived and it became a life-changing moment for the couple as well.

—Jeanne Pernia, PassionLife

3. You are a counselor, so you help her think clearly.

When you are not being directive, you are being facilitative. That is, you're helping her accurately understand her pregnancy. You're educating her about the different options she faces. You're facilitating an internal audit of her own heart values. You're helping her think through the short-term and long-term impacts of her choices. As a counselor, you are there to facilitate wise and healthy decisions.

As you listen, you identify things she doesn't know or misunderstands. These may involve fetal development, abortion procedures and risks, and alternative resources and options. In your role as a counselor, you provide this information and then help her process it in terms of her final decision.

Not all but most women in pregnancy crisis express ambivalence about abortion. In typical cases, the woman hasn't had anyone help her think about why she may be ambivalent in terms of her own values. Your role as a counselor is to help her slow down and understand herself and the reasons for her ambivalence. In this sense, you are a mirror, helping her see what she actually believes and values beneath the pressure of her immediate circumstances.

You are also an echo chamber—restating, clarifying, and amplifying those beliefs. For example, a surprising percentage of women and couples considering abortion will say, "I know abortion is wrong, but I need to do it anyway." You are going to ask her why she thinks it's wrong. Then you are going to clarify her answer in a way that makes it plain for her to understand and easy to hear.

Finally, you are her GPS, helping her to see where her choices may lead "down the road a piece." Each option has outcomes. Each one has hard challenges. But the long-term outcomes are very different. You're there to help her think and understand, perceive her values as well as her circumstances, and then to choose a path that is healthy for her and her unborn child.

4. You are a confidant, so you honor confidentiality.

There are legal and ethical limits to the promise of confidentiality. But before addressing those exceptions, let's address the rule. "In the American Counseling Association (ACA) *Code of Ethics* (2005), counselors are charged with recognizing trust as an important component of the counseling relationship, and they are obligated to facilitate a trusting relationship through the maintenance of client confidentiality."[2] This standard is true no matter what country you live in.

You respect her privacy and honor her by keeping her story, from beginning to end, confidential.[3] Although common sense can usually guide you, in this age of social media, let me say explicitly: confidentiality and social media do not mix. The following is good advice:

> With the popularity and pervasiveness of social media in our everyday lives, it is easy to see how patient privacy can be breached without even realizing it. My rule is to never post messages or comment about work in any way: never post pictures from work and never "friend" any current or past patients via social networking sites.[4]

Should you meet her a year or even several years later, the rule of confidentiality remains in force. I once walked into a store and saw, working at the counter, a young woman who had been in a crisis pregnancy a year earlier. When she saw me, she looked momentarily alarmed. But then our eyes met and said all that needed to be said. I paid for my food and wished her a good day.

If you are doing PCI in the context of a PHO, confidentiality means (apart from peer consultation among the approved staff) that you do not talk about her case with anyone. In that PHO context, remember that the pregnancy test results, the ultrasound confirmation, and whatever else you provide (including what you write down in her client chart), is part of her confidential medical record. In the United States, this record falls under the Health Insurance Portability and Accountability Act (HIPAA). HIPAA regulations (and similar regulations in other countries) are designed to protect patient privacy and safeguard their medical records from becoming public. Also confidential are the notes you make regarding a woman or a couple in a pregnancy-related crisis. A good rule of thumb is never to write down anything you would not want to be seen by the client (woman) or in an open court. Keep your opinions to yourself and learn to keep records in a professional way as your PHO will train you to do.

There are times when you must break confidentiality. In some cases, this is a legal obligation. Teachers, nurses, and licensed counselors are among those designated as "mandated reporters." But even if you're just a friend, there are some confidences that must be broken.

In legal terms, this is usually referred to as *the duty to warn* or *the duty to protect*. For example, if a fourteen-year-old girl tests positive for pregnancy and tells you confidentially that her father is involved, you cannot keep this a secret. The same is true if the man involved with her pregnancy was her twenty-six-year-old math teacher. If she tells you she plans to kill her boyfriend and then herself, that too is not a confidence you can keep. Call the police or appropriate agency immediately.

Pregnancy help organizations have a "Policy and Procedures Manual" and offer specialized training in how to handle confidentiality, recordkeeping, and mandated reporting. Make sure you are familiar with this information. The women coming into a PHO are also provided informed consent regarding their confidentiality. This is usually provided via the intake form that women must sign before meeting with a pregnancy counselor. This form includes a statement regarding confidentiality and assures the woman that her privacy is protected to the extent allowed by law.

In summary, apart from exceptional circumstances that endanger her life or that of others, you want to assure her that what she shares with you is confidential. Assure her that she is in control of her story. Then let her begin to tell it.

As a point of application, this means talking to the women in crisis privately at the beginning, even if she comes in with a parent or boyfriend, and even if she says that they may join you. You use the principle of confidentiality to prevent this. That way you can make an independent assessment of her attitude concerning the pregnancy and of the role others are playing in the crisis.

At a certain point, once you have completed the initial assessment and understand her intentions, it may be wise to expand the conversation to include the significant others who came with her, if she still wants to include them. You are now helping her implement next steps—in this case, communicating her intentions to others or helping her understand the intentions or desires of these significant people in her life.

There will be borderline situations in which you are uncertain about bringing a boyfriend or parent into the circle of discussion. At such times, err on the side of confidentiality until it is clearly the right thing to do.

VOICES FROM THE FIELD

Confidentiality
"Mandated Reporting"

We had a thirteen-year-old present for a pregnancy test. She stated that her boyfriend was thirty years old. She also added, "My mom is okay with it. In fact, she let me move into his house." At this point, I let her know that *I* was *not* okay with it. Her situation was unacceptable—indeed, it was against the law. She was a minor. He was a pedophile. I had no word to describe her mother. The young girl again argued that her mom approved of the situation, and that made it okay. "What if I have her come here and tell you herself?" she asked. "Yes, by all means," I replied. "I'd like to talk to her."

The mother did come to see me. She looked like every other church lady I see on Sunday mornings—not at all what I had envisioned. I asked her what she was thinking, letting her thirteen-year-old daughter live with a thirty-year-old man. She didn't have an answer. I told her that I was going to call the state police. I did and they started an investigation. We went on to refer this minor to professional counseling.

This child was being destroyed by a predator, and her mother was complicit in her daughter's destruction. This girl had no protectors. Mandated reporting laws give you the legal backbone to confront all involved and provide protection from ongoing abuse (and that of others her predator would have targeted). Never hold such things in confidence. Report it immediately to authorities and get a copy of the report and document everything.

—Vikki Parker, Option Pregnancy Center

5. You are a neighbor, so you bring practical help.

Another concept of self-understanding you bring to PCI is that of a neighbor helping a neighbor. A good neighbor is one who helps in direct and practical ways when their neighbor is in a fix.

You are going to make sure she gets a pregnancy test and understands the results. You are going to provide her with accurate medical information regarding her pregnancy and her options. You are going to listen to her vent. You are going to rally her spirit to take the necessary next step. You are going to call her and follow up. You are going to sit with her and make the next appointment or referral.

Over the following days and weeks, you may be calling her numerous times. You may help her talk to her parents or boyfriend. You may check that she has obtained prenatal care. You may develop a parenting plan with her. You may, on occasion, be the person who is with her when she gives birth.

Even highly trained and skilled professionals, such as doctors and lawyers, understand the value of seeing themselves as neighbors helping neighbors. It helps you build relationships. It helps you talk plainly and speak directly. It makes people feel comfortable in speaking with you. It reminds you to be a problem solver. For example, when she says, "What am I going to do?" she's sifting through the next forty years of her projected life. You are thinking practically: What does she need to do *next*? Does she need a pregnancy test? An ultrasound? What does she need to understand about pregnancy and her options? Before she leaves, you need to make sure you have the next step clarified—what she will do tonight or tomorrow. You are the practical one, the good neighbor who helps out in a fix.

6. You are a witness, so you leave the outcome to God.

The pregnancy crisis counselor is a witness to the availability of a life-affirming path forward. You're there to help her take this path. But you cannot make her take it. You may inform, appeal, even caution her about the choices she may make. But having done so in love and good faith, you must respect the nature of things: that each person is created as a moral agent, sovereign over their own choices.

Some people have argued, "If she was about to kill her two-year-old, you would take more compelling steps to stop her. So why not take steps to stop her from killing her two-month-old unborn child?" It is true that there is no morally significant difference between an unborn human being and a two-year-old that justifies killing the unborn while protecting the toddler. What is different is that unborn human beings have been stripped of their legal human rights. Abortion is legal and accessible. The two-year-old is recognized by law as a human being with the full rights afforded to all human beings.

Although abortion is legal in many countries (including the US), this means it is all the more important for you to act as a witness concerning the human dignity of the unborn and make an appeal to the mother to choose life. You are backing up this appeal with the promise of practical help. At that point, your work is done.

If you go beyond your role as a witness, however, then you overstep your boundaries. To clarify what that means, let's state who you are not in the intervention process.

You Are Not the Savior

This is the implication of the point above. You work to educate and persuade. You promise to help. But you also respect God's prerogative to endow every person with moral agency, with the ability to choose for or against his moral law. In saying this, notice we are not using the phrase "freedom to choose." To clarify, God has given people the *ability* to choose between life and death. He has not given them the moral *freedom* to choose between them.

The biblical text to which we allude is italicized in context as found in Deuteronomy 30:15–20. Consider the full text:

> "See, I have set before you today life and good, death and evil. If you obey the commandments of the LORD your God that I command you today, by loving the LORD your God, by walking in his ways, and by keeping his commandments and his statutes and his rules, then you shall live and multiply, and the LORD your God will bless you in the land that you are entering to take possession of it. But if your heart turns away, and you will not hear, but are drawn away to worship other gods and serve them, I declare to you today, that you shall surely perish. You shall not live long in the land that you are going over the Jordan to enter and possess. *I call heaven and earth to witness against you today, that I have set before you life and death, blessing and curse. Therefore choose life,* that you and your offspring may live, loving the LORD your God, obeying his voice and holding fast to him, for he is your life and length of days, that you may dwell in the land that the LORD swore to your fathers, to Abraham, to Isaac, and to Jacob, to give them."

God does not say, "I set before you life and death: *choose one.*" That would be freedom to choose. Rather, he imposes a moral imperative to "choose life" so that in obedience to his law, they would experience a wholeness and fullness of life.

Government authorities do the same thing. They create laws. All laws impose a morality on the community. Laws against robbery or speeding teach that robbery and speeding are wrong in that they rob people of a whole and full life. People have the ability to break these laws. But we never apply the language of "freedom to choose" to things lawfully forbidden. Quite the opposite. You are not free to do these things, though you have the capacity to do them.

In pregnancy crisis intervention, there is a moral appeal to choose life. You may assure her that in choosing life, there is divine blessing and provision. You may promise to be helpful in finding that provision. But you must acknowledge moral agency: the ability to reject life and choose death in spite of your counsel and help. You are not the Savior.

Conclusion

She is in a state of crisis. You, like Job, are willing to intervene: "I was eyes to the blind and feet to the lame. I was a father to the needy, and I searched out the cause of him whom I did not know. I broke the fangs of the unrighteous and made him drop his prey from his teeth" (Job 29:15–17). We turn next to what that intervention looks like when you first meet the woman in crisis.

4

WHEN YOU MEET TOGETHER

*"It is always hard to separate what you really
want from what you're supposed to want."*[1]

—Wendy Shalit

*"Oil and perfume make the heart glad,
and the sweetness of a friend comes from earnest counsel."*

—Proverbs 27:9

By choice or by providence, you're the one she's come to talk to. It matters what you say and do now as you meet together. She alone is responsible for the choice and outcome, but you have influence.

Michaelene is one who turned to a colleague for guidance in the midst of her pregnancy crisis—and she regretted the advice this person gave to her. In the following account, Michaelene presents many of the characteristics of pregnancy crisis that we described in chapter 2. As you read her account, note how the person she turned to for guidance in the midst of her crisis influenced the outcome.

When I became pregnant at 18, my first thought was to have an abortion. The abortion would allow me to continue teaching ballroom dance and training for competition. The idea of adoption did cross my mind. I knew I wasn't ready to parent, but I thought perhaps I could delay my career for the nine months or so that it would take me to carry my baby to term. My 28-year-old live-in boyfriend was furious when he discovered I was pregnant. He immediately demanded that I have an abortion. . . .

I didn't have any other friends or contacts in the area, so I decided to seek advice from the [dance] studio manager. After I told her about my situation, she recommended abortion and offered to arrange one for me. I left the office with the date and the time of the appointment and an arranged ride from my supervisor. . . .

Although I didn't feel this way before the procedure, it was now clear to me that the abortion ended the life of my child. I felt guilty and desired punishment. I deserved to suffer. Afterward, the mere presence of my boyfriend caused deep hurt and pain. I found it difficult to work. . . . I soon found myself in a cycle of self-destructive behavior that included an eating disorder.[2]

It's not difficult to see how a grief-sparing, life-affirming outcome might have developed in this case if the person she turned to for guidance had a clearer understanding of human life and took the time to help Michaelene identify why the adoption option crossed her mind. What were Michaelene's true heart values? And how would aborting her own values (in the abortion itself) affect her afterwards?

This is where you can make a difference when you're the one she turns to in her crisis.

When You Meet Together, What Are Your Goals?

Grief and trauma expert H. Norman Wright says, "In crisis counseling, the person, couple or family must see that they need to make a choice to remain the same or to change and grow. . . . A goal of crisis counseling is to help the person in need accept and take responsibility."[3] In other words, the focus of crisis intervention is not on the precipitating event but on the person needing to adjust, adapt, and grow in response to that event.

In pregnancy crisis counseling, your goal is to help the woman or couple in pregnancy distress find a pathway toward the acceptance of her unborn child and to accept responsibility for developing a parenting plan (or an adoption plan). To do that effectively, you must respond to her crisis with some emotional sensitivity.

Sometimes this is referred to as emotional intelligence (EI). We limit the term to mean only the need for the counselor "to monitor one's own and other people's emotions, to discriminate between different emotions and label them appropriately and to use emotional information to guide thinking and behavior."[4] Simplified for our purposes, it refers to perceiving the presence and controlling the effect of multiple, contrary emotions in the woman or couple before you, so that you can respond to emotion in a life-affirming way.

She may be angry at her partner and feel like punching him. But she may also be so desirous of maintaining a long-term relationship with him that she'll do anything not to lose him, even if that means doing what she doesn't want to do. She may be excited about being pregnant, but she may also desperate not to be. She may feel strong compassion toward the life within her, but she may also fear the intrusion. She may know that her family loves her, but she may also feel embarrassed and ashamed and want to protect them from similar feelings. All of these emotions are present at the same time, and each is vying for control.[5]

With your ultimate goal in mind—helping her find a life-affirming pathway out of the crisis—sit down with her with a series of penultimate goals that address the emotional turmoil she is in.

VOICES FROM THE FIELD

When You Meet Together, What Are Your Goals?
"Emotional Intelligence"

If you are working in a PHO, you will start with an intake sheet, in which the woman will provide some basic medical information and pregnancy history. Even from how she fills out this form, you will gain insight into her state of mind and the dominant emotions of her crisis. When I see that a women fills the sheet with either scribbled, crossed out, or very strong descriptive words, I know there is deep turmoil, mostly anger, brewing inside her.

—Jeanne Pernia, PassionLife

1. She's fearful. You want to lower her fear.

The dominant and controlling emotion in a pregnancy-related crisis is fear. Your goal is to lower this fear. You do this first through your bearing and demeanor, your tone and spirit. Train yourself to speak calmly and be reassuring. A ship in a storm is looking for a calm, strong harbor. You are that harbor.

Even if you're nervous and fearful that you'll say the wrong thing, be self-controlled and keep it to yourself. Be personable—that is, be friendly and interested in the woman or couple. Be professional—relaxed and confident that you can say and do the right thing when it matters most.

Later on in the counseling process, this confident bearing is precisely what you're trying to convey to her. "You can get through this. You're stronger than you know. Things have a way of working out. Don't be afraid. Have faith in yourself and don't compromise your beliefs and values. I will help you. You're not alone."

All such encouragements have the effect of lowering fear and increasing hope. The more her fears go down and her hope rises, the more likely she will take a life-affirming path forward.

2. She's under pressure to abort. You want to give her one reason to resist.

There are many reasons to abort an unborn human being and many immediate benefits. For example, it frees the woman to pursue other things, like a career and financial prosperity. It saves "face." It cleans up the loose ends of a relationship that is ending. It's cheap, fast, and promises instant relief.

There is only one reason that choosing abortion is morally wrong—only one. It's morally wrong to intentionally kill an innocent human being, and abortion intentionally kills an innocent human being. If the unborn is not a human being, then being pregnant presents no greater moral challenge than what to have for dinner or dessert. It's a matter of preference—no different from choosing chocolate or vanilla ice cream. But if the unborn is a human being, then killing him or her to benefit others is morally wrong. It treats the distinct human being, with his or her own inherent moral worth, as nothing more than disposable property. Clearly, if the unborn are human, such as toddlers, we shouldn't kill them in the name of choice any more than we would a two-year-old.

What then is the unborn? Is it human? To answer this question, we turn to science. But science cannot tell us how we ought to treat the unborn. A moral philosophy of human rights must inform our behavior and laws. Scott Klusendorf writes,

> The science of embryology tells us that from the earliest stages of development, the unborn are distinct, living, and whole human beings. Leading embryology books confirm this. For example, Keith L. Moore & T. V. N. Persaud write, "A zygote is the beginning of a new human being. Human development begins at fertilization, the process during which a male gamete or sperm . . . unites with a female gamete or oocyte . . . to form a single cell called a zygote. This highly specialized, totipotent cell marks the beginning of each of us as a unique individual.

Philosophically, we can say that embryos are less developed than newborns (or, for that matter, toddlers). But as Stephen Schwarz points out, there is no morally significant difference between the embryo that you once were and the adult that you are today that would justify killing you at that early stage of development. Differences of size, level of development, environment, and degree of dependency are not relevant such that we can say that you had no rights as an embryo but you do have rights today.[6]

This is the one truth with which a woman under great pressure can defend herself and push back: "You're asking me to kill my own child. I will not do so. Period."

Scott encourages people to think of the acronym "SLED" as a helpful reminder of these nonessential differences:

Size: True, embryos are smaller than newborns and adults, but why is that relevant? Do we really want to say that large people are more human than small ones? Men are generally larger than women, but that doesn't mean that they deserve more rights. Size doesn't equal value.

Level of development: True, embryos and fetuses are less developed than the adults they'll one day become. But again, why is this relevant? Four-year-old girls are less developed than fourteen-year-old ones. Should older children have more rights than their younger siblings? Some people say that self-awareness makes one human. But if that is true, newborns do not qualify as valuable human beings. Six-week-old infants lack the immediate capacity for performing human mental functions, as do the reversibly comatose, the sleeping, and those with Alzheimer's disease.

Environment: Where you are has no bearing on who you are. Does your value change when you cross the street or roll over in bed? If not, how can a journey of eight inches down the birth canal suddenly change the essential nature of the unborn from nonhuman to human? If the unborn are not already human, merely changing their location can't make them valuable.

Degree of Dependency: If viability makes us human, then all those who depend on insulin or kidney medication are not valuable and we may kill them. Conjoined twins who share blood type and bodily systems also have no right to life.

In short, it's far more reasonable to argue that although humans differ immensely with respect to talents, accomplishments, and degrees of development, they are nonetheless equal because they share a common human nature.

The problem is that the humanity of the unborn is vaguely, not clearly, understood by most people. It's not scientifically and philosophically clear enough in their mind to produce the burst of moral courage that would arise, say, if people were pressuring them to terminate their two-year-old to solve the very problems they perceive to be solved by abortion.

To illustrate, Alex was another woman with a crisis pregnancy. Although she knew her unborn was a human being, she didn't quite think her unborn was *as* human as a toddler. She therefore ended up yielding to the pressure the father of her baby put on her:

> I gently reminded him that we were already planning on getting married and that I really couldn't have an abortion. His gentle persistence eventually became more forceful. He tried to convince me that our relationship wouldn't last if I didn't have the abortion. . . .

> My arguments grew weaker until I finally gave in to him. I still didn't want to have the abortion—I knew it would end the life of our child. But I thought that if I got it over with quickly—that if I had the abortion early enough in the pregnancy—then I'd be able to cope with it.[7]

55

Alex knew enough about fetal development to recognize that abortion "would end the life of our child." But absent the clarity of seeing her unborn on ultrasound or having fetal development pictures and models to confirm her beliefs, she rationalized away her own values and yielded.

The truth is that there was no early stage in her pregnancy when Alex's unborn was less human—and no later stage when it would be more human. In her thinking, her unborn was no more a potential human being than a potential frog. But the truth of the matter is that from conception, it is a living, distinct, and whole human being, with lifelong potential.

Your goal is to help her resist the pressure of others by equipping her with the one truth that trumps all the others: her unborn baby is a human being, and she is right to cherish and defend that child's life no matter the hardship—just as she would safeguard her two-year-old.

VOICES FROM THE FIELD

She's Under Pressure
"Lots of People Do Not Know Fetal Science"

One young woman told me that she had already scheduled an abortion when she came to talk to me with her boyfriend. I listened to their fears and hopes. I outlined their options. Then, to help them understand the implications of each option, I took time to examine their baby's fetal development. Their reaction was surprise. They simply did not know about the stage of their baby until that moment. I finished our time together by explaining our pregnancy and parenting education support services, should they carry to term. The next day they came back. They told me that there were two reasons they canceled their abortion appointment. The first was learning the truth about the fetal development of their unborn baby. The second was our pledge to help them navigate a path through their pregnancy and support them through our parenting education services.

—Tina Williams, Alpha Pregnancy Resource Center

3. She sees her pregnancy as life-threatening. You want to help her see a pathway for both her and her baby to live.

Like suicide, abortion is a crisis of faith. Both involve not being able to believe that "things will work out."

Suicide is the wrong way to end a life crisis. Likewise, abortion is also the wrong way to end another life crisis. Both are driven by a despair that makes people feel that they have no choice. Although this is a lie, it *feels* true to that person.

In pregnancy crisis intervention, your goal is to break the lie that tells her she has no choice. She does have a choice. Your goal is to help her find a pathway forward in which she and her unborn child can live. It is true that where there is a will, there is a way. But is that way sacrificial in nature? Sometimes, yes. Good things can come from sacrifice, however, although we may not see that good until we have been willing first to do what is right, no matter what the cost.

To illustrate your goal as a counselor, let's change the context momentarily to a potential suicide. Imagine you come across a jumper. You stop on the bridge to intervene. You may not have time to fully listen and come to know all that has happened in the past that has driven our jumper to the ledge. You certainly don't know how things may work out in the future if he steps back. But you believe things can and will work out, if only he will step back and explore the other options with you or those you will bring to his aid.

A pregnancy-related crisis is likewise a crisis of faith. You may hear, "There is no way I can feed and take care of a baby." This is false. She may not see how, at this moment, she can feed and care for her baby, but the solutions will present themselves in time, if she will only choose life. It happens every day.

Many times I've heard a couple say, "We already have two (or three or four) children. We cannot afford another child." The truth is that they found a way to feed the ones they have. If they lost their jobs in the morning, they would not terminate their kids in the afternoon on the basis of their lowered income and the uncertainty of how to feed and clothe them in the months ahead. They will believe that another way to take care of them will present itself. And it will. Although nobody usually plans for twins or triplets, they do not kill the ones they did not include in their budget. People figure it out as they go.

Listen, then, for statements like, "I want to be a lawyer, and there is no way I can be a lawyer and have a baby." This is not true. Many people have done both. It may mean she can't finish law school in the time frame she planned or without some extra challenges or support. But it can be done, and without sacrificing her baby to accomplish it. Where there is a willingness to choose life, there is a provision for life.

A teen may say, "My parents will kill me." Although this isn't true (at least lawfully in the US), it feels true to her. She is looking at abortion as necessary to save her life. In her mind, it's either "I live or the baby lives." The illogic is self-evident, but the emotions are real. The challenge is to bring perspective to the situation and help her believe that there is life after pregnancy.

4. She wants quick relief. You want to slow things down and help her think.

Norm Wright reminds us that crisis has a short shelf life:

Keep in mind that people cannot tolerate the stress of crisis long. In one way or another, they will resolve it within a period of six weeks. . . . Therefore, many attempts for quick relief that the person makes will not be thought out. They could even be counterproductive by worsening the problems or crisis.[8]

This is especially applicable to pregnancy-related crisis. As David Reardon observed in his study of women after abortion,

> Most of these women indicated that during the time between discovering they were pregnant and having the abortion there was such a high level of emotional trauma that they were unable to thoughtfully and cautiously consider their alternatives. Abortion was simply the most obvious and fastest way to escape from their dilemmas.[9]

After the abortion, not all, but many women report that thinking about the baby is all they can do. The problems that abortion promised to solve merely transform into different and more difficult ones.

Returning to Alex's story, she writes,

> I thought I'd be okay—we'd be okay. I was wrong. I immediately regretted the abortion. I felt the loss of our child from the core of my being. I grieved over my child—our child. I grieved over my inability to stay true to my beliefs. I felt off balance.

> I would cry and he would YELL. Whenever I tried to tell him how I was feeling, he'd storm out. The distance between us kept growing until we finally broke up two months later.

> The loss was unbearable. In fact, the losses were unbearable.[10]

You don't know how the woman sitting with you will respond after the abortion. Some report relief and appear to have little or no regrets. Others experience relief for a while, but after a year or two find themselves sinking into depression and grief. Some are undone almost immediately.

Provide her the opportunity to slow down and consider the testimonies of women such as Alex. As chapter 5 will examine, there are signs of maternal-fetal bonding that are predictors of posttraumatic stress after abortion. What signs does she see? In exploring the different narratives of other women's abortion experiences, she can consider her own reactions thoughtfully. Help her slow down and think this through carefully.

5. She has two minds and hears two voices. You want to help her see why she is ambivalent and amplify the quiet voice of conscience.

The majority of women seeking an abortion don't believe in abortion. As Alex confessed, "I was against abortion, yet I had one."

In our current culture, most women of child-bearing age have been raised to think that sex has little to do with marriage and that abortion is a matter of self-empowerment rather than morality. But the heart does not necessarily agree. It's just cowed into conformity. As Wendy Shalit writes of her generation, "It is always hard to separate what you really want from what you're supposed to want."[11]

This is especially true when it comes to abortion. Your goal in counseling is to help her see what she actually believes about the humanity of her unborn child and why she is "against abortion" even as she is considering it. You're not telling her what you believe. You're helping her listen to the voice of her own conscience. You're helping her identify and express her own values.

Most of the time, if you listen carefully, a woman in crisis pregnancy will tell you how to save her baby, if it can be saved. She will express her own ambivalence. Some say it plainly, "I don't want one, but I must have one." Others say it more subtly. So listen carefully.

For example, some time ago, I met with a graduate school student. She spent an unusual amount of time making a list of all the reasons why she needed an abortion and shared them with me. It became clear that with each reason, she was expecting my affirmation. But I simply listened, so she kept adding to her list.

As we saw earlier in this chapter, if the unborn is not human, then no list is needed. If it is a human, then no list of reasons will justify taking the child's life.

When I finally realized this grad student was building a case, I said to her, "You've made quite a list of good reasons why you need an abortion. It seems like you really want me to agree with you that this is the right thing to do. Why is that?"

She replied, "I just want you to know who I really am. I am really a very caring and compassionate person. In fact, I once had a dog and when I moved, I couldn't take the dog with me. So I found a home for it."

It took a long time, but she finally told me how to save her and her unborn child. She was trying to reconcile her self-image as an extremely caring person with her plans to abort her child. She needed my help. In truth, these two cannot be reconciled. Her self-image and her unborn will both live or die together. They are connected by an umbilical cord that is psychological, emotional, and spiritual, as well as physical.

I responded, "If being a kind and caring person is so central to who you are that you placed your dog for adoption, then perhaps you might stay true to who you really are and treat your unborn the way you treated your dog? Find a home for your unborn child. Then you will feel proud of how you handled this situation, just as you're proud of how you took care of your dog."

After a thoughtful pause, she said, "I can do that."

In this case, all I did was help her listen to the quiet voice of her own heart, not the worldly voice that was trying to convince her to go against her own conscience. I listened, and she finally showed me how to help her choose life. Then I simply encouraged her to follow the voice of her own sense of right and wrong, no matter what difficulties might arise—to be the woman of character she really was.

She Has Two Minds
"I Can't Have A Baby/I Can't Abort!"

Jazmin was a 4.0 GPA student and had just received a full scholarship for college. She was young and ambitious and then suddenly pregnant. Her mother's disappointment was so great that she told her to get an abortion or leave the house. As she lay on the table at the abortion clinic, she felt waves of anguish over what she was about to do. She begged the nurse to show her the ultrasound. The nurse told her there was nothing to see. She started crying and told the nurse she had to leave. The nurse told her they would not return her money. Still, she got dressed and left.

Jazmin called a friend who brought her to our PHO. When we did the ultrasound, Jazmin saw her tiny baby of twelve weeks fully formed. She wanted her baby. Her mother and her boyfriend refused all pleas, so she decided to go back for the abortion. But she couldn't do it. Nor could she go home.

We found her a home to stay in. Two months later, her boyfriend asked for forgiveness and pledged his support. Baby Isabella was born. Jazmin and her mother restored their relationship, and Jazmin obtained her bachelor's degree. But what a battle she endured within herself and within her family.

—Martha Avila, Heartbeat of Miami

6. She feels alone. You want to promise to walk with her through the crisis.

Pregnancy is normally the creative work of two people.[12] Raising a child is no different. To do it alone feels both unnatural and impossible. It's not impossible for a single mom, but it does mean doing the work of two. Many mothers, of course, find the strength to do the work of both parents out of necessity. The father of the child has been torn away by tragedy—or, most likely, by immaturity and irresponsibility.

For many women in a pregnancy-related crisis, the sense of being alone is the deciding factor, in spite of what they truly want and truly believe is the right thing to do. As Cheryl says, "If I had one person rallying to my side, I could have had my baby. . . . [I]f I had one person say, 'Cheryl, don't do that. Leave this jerk' . . . I would have done it in a minute."[13] But she didn't have that one person.

You can be that one person that proves she is not alone. Your goal is to communicate simply, "You're not alone. *Together*, we will find a life-affirming pathway out of this crisis."

7. She feels hopeless. You want to increase her hope that things will work out.

Pregnancy crisis intervention as a whole is about lowering fear and raising hope. It involves a lot of listening and educating, and examining of values and beliefs. It involves practical help and, at times, some long-term monitoring and mentoring. All of this activity comes down to lowering fear and increasing hope.

You may speak hopefully in general terms, but exploring matters of faith is also entirely appropriate. This is not just true because of your personal convictions that God exists and can be trusted to provide for a child he created. It's true because most likely the woman or couple before you has been "praying" and is wrestling with their faith as a result of the crisis.

Exploring matters of faith is inherently a large part of crisis and crisis resolution. In the standard (secular) textbook *Crisis Intervention Strategies* (now in its eighth edition and used in universities in general), Richard James and Burl Gilliland forthrightly state:

Faith plays a huge role in the outcome of a crisis as people attempt to make sense of events that seemingly make no sense at all. Faith plays a large part in how people try to come to terms with a randomly cruel universe that crashes down on the notion of a supreme being that runs a just and moral world.[14]

Therefore, exploring matters of faith is not only appropriate, it's crucial in most cases. James and Gilliland further write,

To deny or act as if religion, faith, or spirituality are not part of any crisis is to neglect a large part of a crisis response for most people. Exclusive of pastoral counseling, it is interesting that little space is given to the effects that religion has in the counseling business. Yet for most people trauma is the ultimate challenge to meaning making, and for most people, that meaning making is attached to some kind of faith.[15]

People in crisis are usually praying people. The woman before you will most likely say that she believes in God and then proceed to tell you about her religious background. While she may be off the path, she knows the path is there. She may have been sexually active under conditions that violate her religious ethics. But that same religion tells her that only God can create a baby. She may be considering abortion yet asking God for forgiveness at the same time.

So go ahead and open up the topic. What does her faith say? Who made her baby? Where is God in her life? Can she turn (return) to him? What does she think God's will is right now? Can he be trusted and obeyed? Would she like you to share one or two of the promises in the Bible that may help her at this time?

If these are not relevant questions in her mind, then move on. Obviously, this area of conversation must be handled like all other areas—with maturity and respect, and with her expressed consent. Most often, however, the woman or couple in pregnancy distress welcomes the question, "Tell me about your faith. Where is God in this crisis?"

She Feels Hopeless
"Explore Matters of Faith"

Having understood a woman's difficult circumstances, we also want to understand what is happening "spiritually." Most women do have religious beliefs, and God is very much an active voice or thought for them in their crisis.

Sharon was forty-seven years old when she came to our clinic. She had taken a pregnancy test at home and it was positive. But she said she was going through the "change" and there was no way she could be pregnant at her age. If she was pregnant, then she wanted an abortion. She already had two other children, one away in college and a son in high school. "I'm too old to start again," she said. In addition, her husband would leave her if she even thought about keeping this pregnancy. We then asked about her faith and beliefs. She opened up, and I too shared openly with her about what my own faith says: that even if her husband left her, God would never leave her nor forsake her.

Then we went in together for her ultrasound. Sharon was twenty-two weeks pregnant with triplets and they were all boys! Suddenly, from thinking she was in menopause to wanting an abortion, to being afraid of her husband leaving her, she exclaimed, "*God* has blessed my womb!" and "It's a miracle!" Dylan, Denere, and Denard were born healthy and strong. Given her age and lack of fertility treatments, the doctors called them a miracle too. Sharon considers herself "very blessed." She testifies that "God has provided" for her.

—Martha Avila, Heartbeat of Miami

What is more, people with little faith, or a faith that has been lost or buried under years of regretful decisions, will welcome words of hope. Provide a few.

The LORD takes pleasure in those who fear him,
> in those who hope in his steadfast love.
(Psalm 147:11)

There are many who have prayed for help in the day of crisis. Offer her this prayer to God:

Turn to me and be gracious to me,
> for I am lonely and afflicted.
The troubles of my heart are enlarged;
> bring me out of my distresses.
Consider my affliction and my trouble,
> and forgive all my sins. (Psalm 25:16–18)

God promises to work things out for good if we call upon him in our trouble.

For he delivers the needy when he calls,
> the poor and him who has no helper.
He has pity on the weak and the needy,
> and saves the lives of the needy.
From oppression and violence he redeems their life,
> and precious is their blood in his sight.
(Psalm 72:12–14)

Those who trust in God and obey his commands find direction and new life.

My soul melts away for sorrow;
> strengthen me according to your word!
Put false ways far from me
> and graciously teach me your law!
I have chosen the way of faithfulness;
> I set your rules before me.

I cling to your testimonies, O LORD;
  let me not be put to shame!
I will run in the way of your commandments
  when you enlarge my heart! (Psalm 119:28–32)

Jesus teaches us to hope in God and look to him for our daily needs, saying.

"Therefore I tell you, do not be anxious about your life, what you will eat or what you will drink, nor about your body, what you will put on. . . . Look at the birds of the air: they neither sow nor reap nor gather into barns, and yet your heavenly Father feeds them. Are you not of more value than they?" (Matthew 6:25–26)

He tells us the real secret to feeding ourselves and our families: ask God.

"Pray then like this:

  'Our Father in heaven,
  hallowed be your name.
  Your kingdom come,
  your will be done,
    on earth as it is in heaven.
  Give us this day our daily bread.' " (Matthew 6:9–11)

Do not feel pressured to share any of these promises or to offer your prayers of support. But do not be embarrassed or fearful either. In regard to "religion," James and Gilliland acknowledge,

Many human services workers regard it as an exposed electrical wire, not to be touched on pain of death for fear they will be seen as either proselytizing for their religion or insensitive to other spiritual beliefs[;] however, to deny or act as if religion, faith and spirituality are not part of any crisis is to neglect a large part of a crisis response for most people.[16]

Do not worry about what others say or may say in our increasingly secular culture. In your defense, you have the American Psychological Association. It recommends exploring the religious values of women considering abortion, for they have a higher risk of experiencing negative reactions and trauma after abortion.

> A woman who regards abortion as conflicting with her own and her family's deeply held religious, spiritual, or cultural beliefs but who nonetheless decides to terminate an unplanned or unwanted pregnancy may appraise that experience as more stressful than would a woman who does not regard an abortion as in conflict with her own values or those of others in her social network.[17]

Be true to yourself and do what is best for the woman in crisis before you. Lower her fears. Raise her hope.

With these goals in mind for meeting together, you will want to know the order of the intervention process. But first, I think it best to take something of a deep dive and examine the legal principles and the scientific research that informs the most difficult part of the intervention process: talking openly and honestly about abortion itself.

GROUNDING YOUR COUNSELING IN INFORMED CONSENT

"To offer an unbiased and valid synopsis of the scientific literature on increased risks of abortion, the information must include depression, substance abuse, and anxiety disorders, including Post Traumatic Stress Disorder (PTSD), as well as suicide ideation and behaviors."[1]

—Priscilla Coleman, PhD

Whoever speaks the truth gives honest evidence.

—Proverbs 12:17

How do we talk truthfully about abortion with women in a pregnancy-related crisis? Why is it ethically required of us to inform people considering abortion about the physical and mental health risks associated with it? As counselors, how should we raise disquieting questions and provide accurate, science-based answers?

The Legal Basis for PCI

Within the field of medicine, ethicists have created the legal justification for medical treatment. It's called "informed consent."

The phrase "informed consent" was first used in US case law in 1957.[2] The US President's Commission for the Study of Ethical Problems in Medicine and Biomedical and Behavioral Research (1982) examines the history and development of the "doctrine of informed consent."[3] This doctrine, or principle, was developed to ensure that the metaphysical values of human dignity, autonomy, and moral agency are respected by medical providers. Whether you are a volunteer counselor at a PHO or merely a concerned friend at a coffee shop, the principle of informed consent is what justifies talking truthfully about abortion and raising the uncomfortable question, "What might go wrong?"

Informed consent requires that the person considering a medical treatment has the mental capacity to understand and agree.[4] The two basic elements of informed consent are truthtelling and consent-seeking. In practical terms, informed consent means educating people by using accurate and understandable descriptions of the medical procedures under consideration and the health risks associated with them. It also means ensuring that the person's consent to medical treatment is made without coercion or manipulation.

The principle of informed consent is not part of the moral/political divide over elective abortion. Consider the medical textbook *Management of Unintended and Abnormal Pregnancy: Comprehensive Abortion Care*. This textbook, dedicated to "abortion providers through the world" and endorsed by the National Abortion Federation, states:

Informed consent must include three elements: (1) patients must *have the capacity to make decisions* about their care; (2) their participation in these decisions must be *without coercion or manipulation*; and (3) patients must *be given appropriate information* germane to making the particular decision. The goal of the informed consent process is to protect personal well-being and individual autonomy by providing information on the procedure, risks, and alternatives to the medical intervention being considered.[5]

Grounding your counseling in the principle of informed consent not only justifies educating women and couples considering abortion about the possible negative physical and emotional consequences (called "sequela" in the research, which is the secondary result or the aftereffect), it obligates us to do so. Informed consent makes it inappropriate to withhold information from women considering abortion. Just because the information may be uncomfortable to hear or arouse feelings of discomfort, this does not negate a person's right to know before consenting. All surgical procedures, when shown or explained, have disquieting elements. All medical treatments have negative risks, however small, that can raise fears. The principle of informed consent says that adults must be informed of these risks and then determine their treatment plan.

The Canadian Medical Association (CMA) Code of Ethics makes the following recommendations:

> Provide your patients with the information they need to make informed decisions about their medical care, and answer their questions to the best of your ability.

> Make every reasonable effort to communicate with your patient in such a way that information exchanged is understood.

> Recommend only those diagnostic and therapeutic services that you consider to be beneficial to your patient or to others. If a service is recommended for the benefit of others, as for example in matters of public health, inform your patient of this fact and proceed only with explicit informed consent or where required by law.

> Respect the right of a competent patient to accept or reject any medical care recommended.[6]

In summary, your obligation in PCI is to tell the truth about abortion in a sensitive and patient way. Specifically, explain the kind of abortion procedure she will undergo given her stage of pregnancy. Review the evidenced-based negative outcomes associated with that procedure and the degree of risk, where possible. Finally, as the Code of Ethics says, you are not obligated to recommend an option that you do not believe is in her best interest. Recommend only those options you think are in the best interest of the woman—a life-affirming option.

The Scientific Basis for PCI

If the doctrine of informed consent provides you with a sound *legal* basis for talking honestly about abortion, then the science of maternal-fetal attachment (MFA) provides you with a sound *scientific* basis for talking about it.[7]

MFA refers to the "emotional tie or bond that normally develops between the pregnant woman and her unborn infant."[8] It refers to the affiliation and interaction between them. MFA expresses itself in both emotions and behaviors, such as patting the stomach or talking to the unborn child.

Published literature finds that this bond between a mother and her child starts *in utero*, not at birth. Over seventy years of research, involving women from many countries and diverse cultures, confirm that MFA is a universal experience. Some women report having a sense of attachment very early in their pregnancy, soon after conception. More recent studies have examined the biological basis for MFA: the presence of the hormone oxytocin.

> Oxytocin is a powerful hormone that acts as a neurotransmitter in the brain. It regulates social interaction and sexual reproduction, playing a role in behaviors from maternal-infant bonding and milk release to empathy, generosity, and orgasm. When we hug or kiss a loved one, oxytocin levels increase; hence, oxytocin is often called "the love hormone."[9]

It's useful and even critical for our task as counselors to realize that MFA is present even when there is the intention of abortion. Australian researchers S. Allanson and J. Astbury interviewed women at an abortion clinic and found that 40 percent of those intending abortion talked to their unborn child and 30 percent identified as having "patted my tummy affectionately."[10] In a Swedish study of 499 women requesting first-trimester induced abortion, 67 percent identified as feeling attached to the baby prior to their abortion.[11] One woman wrote, "Immediately when I found out I was pregnant, I felt like a mother. It felt like I had some kind of affinity with the child, and now afterwards, it feels empty." Additionally, "almost 50% of women reported a need for special acts in relation to the abortion." These acts included lighting a candle for the child and asking for forgiveness.

A British study examined abortion in women at menopause. The study revealed that some women had long-lasting attachment to the child lost to abortion many years previously. One woman, Elaine, said, "This child of mine would have been [number of years] this month," referring to the expected due date she had been given for her pregnancy. "I still think about this baby. . . . I don't think I'll ever forget it if I live to be a hundred."[12]

Seeing one's unborn child increases MFA significantly. Ultrasound brings unclear thoughts and feelings regarding the unborn into concrete reality. The impact of seeing one's unborn child on ultrasound can have an immediate effect on a woman's intention to abort. This became clear from the earliest days of ultrasound. In a 1983 study, "Maternal Bonding in Early Ultrasound Fetal Examinations," published in the *New England Journal of Medicine*, Drs. John Fletcher and Mark Evans write,

> One of us pointed to the small, visibly moving fetal form on the screen and asked, "How do you feel about seeing what is inside you?" She answered crisply, "It certainly makes you think twice about abortion." When asked to say

more, she told of the surprise she felt on viewing the fetal form, especially on seeing it move: "I feel that it is human. It belongs to me. I couldn't have an abortion now."[13]

In my own experience, ultrasound's impact is not so great that it changes the intentions of all women intending abortion. But with some, it does have immediate and dramatic impact in bonding a mother to her unborn child. In one case, a couple came into our PHO fully intending abortion. The ultrasound exam, in this case, was indicated to confirm an intact uterine pregnancy and the gestational age (that, in turn, indicates which abortion procedure would be used, which is information they need to understand as part of informed consent). On screen, the baby kicked several times. The mother exclaimed, "Look, our baby is a soccer player!" It appeared that her spoken intention to terminate the pregnancy had not only changed, but it also was forgotten.

On the other hand, substance abuse, depression, a domineering partner, a lack of family or social support all inhibit MFA. You don't have to be a trained professional to perceive that a mother having a baby while taking drugs will endanger her child *in utero* and that the child is at a greater risk of neglect or violence.

Most important relative to pregnancy crisis intervention is to know that *the degree of bonding established during pregnancy is predictive of the degree of emotional distress and trauma symptoms experienced after the abortion.*

VOICES FROM THE FIELD

Maternal-Fetal Attachment and Ultrasound
"Bonded through Ultrasound"

Carley, the mother of an eight-month-old son, found out she was pregnant. Although she had always been against abortion, she stated, "I'm out of work and can barely take care of my son. There's no way I can care for another baby. I have no choice but to abort." But after seeing her nine-week baby on ultrasound, everything changed. Upon seeing her unborn child, she felt an immediate and deep bond. With our commitment to help her, she resolved, "I'm just going to find a way."

—Peggy Benicke, Robbinsdale Women's Center

Negative Emotional Reactions and Posttraumatic Stress Disorder (PTSD) after Abortion

PTSD, also called PTS, is a clinically defined term with specific diagnostic criteria.[14] Dr. Martha Shuping explains,

> PTSD is a disorder that by definition starts with a traumatic event. The trauma is not just any unpleasant event, but "exposure to actual or threatened death, serious injury, or sexual violence" (American Psychiatric Association, 2013). Examples could include witnessing a child being hit by a car, or experiencing combat situation in which you were in danger of death. In the case of abortion, if a woman has started thinking of the fetus as her own child prior to the abortion, she may then experience the abortion as the death of her child, which is one predictor for the possible development of PTSD. Not all women develop PTSD after abortion, but there is evidence that some do.[15]

A Clinician's Guide to Medical and Surgical Abortion is a textbook written by and for abortion providers. In the section on the psychological reactions after abortion, they list "negative reactions."[16] These negative reactions include symptoms of PTSD defined trauma:

> Suicidal ideation, losing interest in enjoyable activities . . . interpreting any misfortune, illness, or accident as signs of God's punishment; having nightmares about killing or

saving babies; engaging in self-punishing behaviors such as substance abuse, indiscriminate sex, and relationships with abusive partners; blocking out the experience; and avoiding anything that triggers memories of the event . . . relentless thoughts of being a bad person . . . engaging in thoughts or behaviors that perpetuate a strong emotional investment in the pregnancy or that prevent the redirection of emotional energy into moving forward with life.

In spite of this acknowledgment, researchers Angela Lanfranchi, Ian Gentles, and Elizabeth Ring-Cassidy report,

The question of abortion's psychological impact on women is highly contested in the social science literature. . . . Because of the highly controversial nature of the mental-health consequences of abortion, it is extremely difficult to carry out objective, scientific research in this area. As in other areas, such as climate change or nutrition, once a politically correct position has been established, any publications that challenge that position tend to be ignored, dismissed or undermined.[17]

Sadly, as Lanfranchi et al. point out, there is even a bias in thinking about bias:

Those authors who publish results that challenge the prevailing position that abortion does not cause negative psychological impacts are accused of having an anti-abortion agenda. Those whose research supports the status quo, on the other hand, are characterized as "independent" scientists. In the area of psychological outcomes after abortion, no pro-abortion bias is ever identified or even suggested in the mainstream literature.[18]

Australia's University of Adelaide scholar Erica Millar writes in *Happy Abortions: Our Bodies in the Era of Choice*, "From the perspective of the unwilling pregnant woman, we can see abortion as something to be celebrated rather than a choice to be tolerated."[19] She emphasizes the sense of relief (happiness) that many, though not all, women experience immediately following abortion. For example, Amelia Bonow writes of her experience: "Abortion made me happy in a totally unqualified way. Why wouldn't I be happy that I was not forced to become a mother?"[20]

How are we to account then for the chronic guilt, grief, and depression reported by women in their own abortion experience narratives? Millar argues that pro-life activists are to blame for creating an "emotional script" surrounding abortion. She claims that the anguish, shame, grief, and self-destructive behaviors associated with abortion-related PTSD are caused by anti-abortion narratives, not the abortion itself. Millar concludes that "abortion carries no predictable acute or prolonged emotional or mental health consequences for women."[21] To reach this conclusion, you must choose your studies carefully and ignore many others.

More nuanced is the Task Force on Mental Health and Abortion of the American Psychological Association. Their report concluded that "the relative risk of mental health problems among adult women who have a single, legal, first-trimester abortion of an unwanted pregnancy for nontherapeutic reasons is no greater than the risk of women who deliver an unwanted pregnancy."[22]

Those unfamiliar with sociological research and methodological limitations are apt to conclude that the APA Task Force is agreeing with Millar's assertion that "abortion carries no predictable acute or prolonged emotional or mental health consequences for women." Psychiatrist and PTSD expert Martha Shuping clarifies the statement:

This conclusion applies only to women in these subgroups:

- Adult women, age 21 and above (excludes 18% of U.S. abortion patients who are teens; Jones, Finer, and Singh, 2010).

- Single abortion—not repeats (excludes about half of U.S. abortions; Cohen, 2007).

- First-trimester abortion (excludes 11% of U.S. abortions, which are late-term; Guttmacher Institute, 2014).

- Unwanted pregnancy (excludes the pressured/coerced and ambivalent, prevalence unknown).

- Nontherapeutic reasons (excludes those terminating due to medical reasons).

Thus, the conclusion applies to only a minority of women having abortions. More than half of U.S. abortion patients are excluded.[23]

Since more than half of US abortions are not included in the APA finding, Shuping concludes that it is "not helpful in establishing whether abortion can be traumatic. *It is widely accepted that PTSD occurs only in a percentage of those exposed to any trauma.*"[24]

In 1988, Congress ordered the National Vietnam Veteran's Readjustment Study (NVVRS) in order to identify the prevalence of PTSD in American veterans of the war in Vietnam. Shuping writes,

In the NVVRS, lifetime prevalence of PTSD—veterans who had ever suffered—was 30.9% for full PTSD and 22.5% for partial PTSD (Kulka et al., 1988; Price, 2015). Thus, the majority of combat veterans did not meet full criteria for PTSD, though slightly more than half, 53%, had at least some symptoms over their lifetimes. At the time of the study only 15.2% of male combat veterans had current full PTSD. Similarly, the National Women's Study showed 31% of women who were raped have PTSD symptoms at some time afterwards, with 11% still having it currently (Kilpatrick, 2000). Thus, a majority of combat veterans and a majority of rape survivors did not meet diagnostic criteria for full PTSD. Yet PTSD in these groups is still considered a substantial clinical problem meriting attention.[25]

Researchers on both sides of the moral/political divide regarding elective abortion acknowledge that some women under specific circumstances report no negative effects after their abortion. A percentage of women report positive feelings of relief. From the crisis management perspective, this is expected. People can live in a state of crisis only for a short time before something will be done to relieve it.

The larger issue is whether abortion, having ended the immediate pregnancy crisis, impacts a percentage of women in traumatic or unhealthy ways. What is the scope of mental health issues and what is the prevalence suffered?

Examining abortion-related PTSD, the deVeber Institute for Bioethics and Social Research sifted through 650 extensively researched and published papers in medical and psychological journals. The researchers, Lanfranchi et al., provide their conclusions in *Complications: Abortion's Impact on Women*. Regarding the psychological and social impact of abortion, they conclude that "the increase in the rate of depression, anxiety, substance abuse and suicide among women who have had an abortion is drastic and incontrovertible."[26] Further, " *We are more than ever persuaded of the urgency of communicating this information to medical professionals, counselors, and to women who are contemplating having an abortion.*"[27]

They point to the meta-analysis research of Priscilla Coleman as especially weighty.[28] Coleman identified twenty-two studies published between 1995 and 2009 that used a sample size of at least one hundred women. Coleman's methods, criteria, and controls were sufficient to have her research published in the peer-reviewed *British Journal of Psychiatry* in 2011. Though her work was attacked soon after, the journal stood behind it: "Her review of these studies strongly supported an association between abortion and mental health problems.

She discovered an overall 81 percent greater risk of mental health problems for women who had an abortion compared to those who did not."[29]

In her article, Coleman summarized the type of risks and the increased risk percentage as follows:

1. Anxiety disorders—34%
2. Depression—37%
3. Alcohol use/abuse—110%
4. Marijuana use/abuse—220%
5. Suicide behaviors—155%[30]

Lanfranchi and the others review of PTSD after abortion says that "the weight of evidence supports the conclusion that for a significant minority of women abortion has a devastating long-term psychological impact."[31] Elaine's abortion narrative is a case in point: "I was just so depressed, I didn't want to live anymore, I was suicidal and I started drinking, because all I could think about is that I've murdered this baby." Looking back on her abortion experience, she said it affected her "a lot more than I ever thought it would."[32]

VOICES FROM THE FIELD

Negative Reactions
"Delayed PTSD"

The psychiatric diagnostic manual *DSM-5* (American Psychiatric Association, 2013) says that some people who develop PTSD may do so with "delayed expression," when the criteria for the diagnosis of PTSD are not met until more than six months after a traumatic event. In some cases, women may have experienced no prior attachment to the unborn child and yet later events, such as seeing the ultrasound of their first *intended* child, may change their perception of the previously aborted fetus and the woman may experience PTSD symptoms that emerge at that time. For example, Kay Lyn Carlson writes that she didn't allow herself to have thoughts or feelings about the baby before the abortion, though later she felt love for her child and deep grief:

> At seventeen, the second I found out I was pregnant, I started making plans to have an abortion. I was in crisis. My dad had once told me that if I ever got pregnant that he would kick me out of the house so fast and cut off all support. I believed him so I didn't allow myself to think or feel anything about the baby, only the task ahead of me. The night before the abortion I went out drinking with my friends. I remember feeling sad and shameful about consuming alcohol and reasoned, "Well, I'm going to kill the baby anyway tomorrow, so what does it matter?" Little did I know at the time how much I would later love and deeply grieve the loss of my child.

Kay Lyn also reported the symptoms that she experienced later, including disturbing dreams, intrusive memories, and other symptoms of PTSD.

—Martha Shuping, MD, Psychiatrist

Informed Consent, MFA, and PTSD after Abortion

The woman you are talking to might never experience anything as destructive as Elaine's experience after her abortion. It is possible she may experience relief similar to Amelia Bonow as reported in *Happy Abortions*. Grounding your counseling in informed consent means informing her of narratives like Elaine's. Screen her for the risk factors predictive of after-abortion trauma or full PTSD.

Even those who strongly oppose the work of PHOs and advocate for elective abortion recognize the need to screen for PTSD after abortion. The 2009 textbook *Management of Unintended and Abnormal Pregnancy: Comprehensive Abortion*

Care lists eighteen "Risk Factors for Negative Emotional Sequelae"[33] and provides a "needs assessment form" for use in counseling women intending abortion.

The following assessment tool provides the counselor a way to help a woman considering abortion identify her predisposing factors for emotional stress and trauma after abortion.

Risk Factors for Negative Emotional Sequelae

- Appraisal of abortion as extremely stressful before it occurs

- Experiencing social stigma and anti-abortion demonstrations on the day of the abortion

- An existing emotional disorder or mental illness prior to the abortion

- Significant ambivalence about the decision

- Perceived coercion to have the abortion

- Intense guilt and shame before the abortion

- Belief that abortion is the same act as killing a newborn infant

- Lack of emotional support and receiving criticism from significant people in their lives

- Fetal abnormality or other medical indications for the abortion

- Commitment and attachment to the pregnancy

- Advance stage of pregnancy

- Putting great effort into keeping the abortion a secret for fear of stigma

- Usual coping style is denial and repressing thoughts

- Unresolved past losses and perception of abortion as a loss

- Past or present sexual, physical, or emotional abuse

- Preexisting experience of trauma

- Expecting depression, severe grief or guilt, and regret after the abortion

- Disbelief in their ability to do what it takes to produce a positive outcome[34]

Voices from the Field

Negative Reactions
"Dreams of Saving Babies"

Just as the MFA (maternal-fetal attachment) research shows, my sense of attachment and loss continues decades after my abortions. And just as the *Clinicians Guide* textbook says, my own negative reactions to abortion have included dreams about saving babies.

Although my abortions happened over forty years ago, I still have occasional dreams about saving babies that are in dangerous situations—for example, on the floor of a public restroom. I don't remember how far along I was when I aborted, but the babies in my dreams always fit in the palm of my hand. I'm always amazed because they are as alert as a much older infant would be, sometimes even crawling on the floor. In my dreams, I cradle and comfort them, feeling great relief that they are safe.

—Peggy Benicke, Robbinsdale Women's Center

Three of the risk factors identified in this list deserve special comment, which are discussed below. They point to predisposing factors you will typically see when counseling women or couples in a pregnancy-related crisis.

1. "Commitment and attachment to the pregnancy"

This factor is an acknowledgment that maternal-fetal bonding is a major predictor for PTSD. In my twenty-five years of work in PCI, more often than not, women considering abortion express a maternal-fetal attachment to some degree. "I don't believe in abortion, but I need one anyway" probably best summarizes the ambivalence of feelings created by a sense of attachment. Sometimes this sense of attachment is so strong that a woman will, rubbing her stomach, apologize to her unborn child for intending to abort. As Shuping stated, "The degree of bonding that is established during pregnancy is predictive of the degree of emotional distress and trauma symptoms that are experienced after the abortion."

2. "Belief that abortion is the same act as killing a newborn infant"

A woman's sense of the humanity of her unborn child is a major risk factor for PTSD. The more a woman sees her pregnancy through the lens of biological truth and religious teaching regarding the humanity of the unborn child, the more her abortion is a termination of her own values and beliefs. Such women are at a higher risk for immediate PTSD. Indeed, researchers Mufel, Speckhard, and Sivuha conclude,

> Attachment to the fetus/embryo and recognition of life are the strongest and most prevalent predictors of adverse psychological responses to abortion for all of the variables examined. . . . In our estimation this reflects standard posttraumatic stress theory that individual perception of a traumatic stressor is the defining issue. Hence, whether or not society views abortion as involving the death of a human being is less important than the woman's own views of the event. When an abortion is perceived by the woman as involving a human death event, and one of a being to who one is related (i.e. "my child") it can act as a traumatic stressor capable of causing PTSD as well as clinically significant responses of guilt, grief and depression.[35]

As a counselor, it is not important for me to tell her my views of abortion. It is important that I help her identify and express her own views. As the training manual *A Clinician's Guide to Medical and Surgical Abortion* advises, her "belief that a fetus is the same as a 4-year-old and that abortion is murder," or her expressed conviction that "abortion is killing a baby," provides the opportunity to help her perceive and predict how she will react later.[36]

Ask, "How do you think you will feel afterwards?" Be prepared to validate her answer by providing her information related to guilt, grief, or PTSD after abortion. Now is also a good time to again express empathy: "I can see now why you are in such terrible anguish." Then ask, "Before you do what you believe so strongly is wrong, would you like to look at some other options?"

3. "Perceived coercion to have the abortion"

The pressure imposed on a woman to abort is a major risk factor for PTSD. If she is being threatened or coerced, or if she *perceives* that she is being manipulated into doing what she does not truly want to do, then she is exposed to a much higher risk of trauma after the abortion.[37] In these cases, the woman is yielding her values and desires to others. It is understandable that anger, grief, regret, and depression may follow. Consider Mandy's testimony:

> My boyfriend did not change his opinion with regards to my pregnancy: I was to have an abortion. . . . A doctor joined and he too said: "It is better to have it done. . . . [T]he father does not want it." I was not to think about myself, not to be selfish. . . . When I finally got the strength to get up and leave, I felt broken.[38]

Because you are a counselor, the doctrine of informed consent directs you to look for outside pressure and, if need be, shield her from these pressures to the degree possible. In one case, I had to call the police to escort her home and then to a shelter to protect her from intimate partner violence. In most cases, it means sitting down with the father of the child on a second visit or meeting with parents.

Conclusion

As we have seen in this chapter, the duty of care in pregnancy crisis intervention is summarized as "informed consent." Informing women of the physical, emotional, psychological, familial, and spiritual risks associated with abortion is the substance of informed consent. In the context of a PHO, this information will be readily available. While the science is politicized and results highly contested, we have seen where there is common ground. In any event, the principle of informed consent provides a solid basis for an honest discussion of the research.

6

UNDERSTANDING PREGNANCY CRISIS INTERVENTION AS A PROCESS

"She really encouraged me and showed me that I could have my baby. I wouldn't have my baby today if it wasn't for her."

—Charis

*For by you I can run against a troop,
and by my God I can leap over a wall.*

—Psalm 18:29

Crisis intervention unfolds like a novel.

No two novels are alike. The people in each, with their particular blend of character and motives, history and happenstance, are unique to that story. Yet all novels share a basic structure: a compelling introduction, a sympathetic protagonist, a building conflict, and a final resolution.

In the same way, pregnancy crisis is idiosyncratic, arising from the unique combination of personalities and character that make up a woman's own story. No two interventions, then, will be the same. Yet all crisis intervention shares a basic structure in terms of having recognizable phases and transition points.

Douglas Puryear, in his book *Helping People in Crisis*, provides one way to map these phases, outlining a seven-step approach for intervention:[1]

Step 1. Establishing communication and rapport
Step 2. Assessing the problem
Step 3. Assessing the resources and strengths
Step 4. Formulating a plan
Step 5. Mobilizing the client
Step 6. Closing
Step 7. Follow-up

As a general map for all kinds of crisis intervention, this is a good start. Norm Wright speaks of Basic Intervention Procedures (BIPs) and suggests using the grief model proposed by Joanne Jozefowski as a guide for crisis intervention,[2] whose model is nearer to that commonly used in the field of pregnancy intervention:

1. Listen
2. Assess
3. Normalize
4. Reassure
5. Support
6. Plan
7. Educate
8. Monitor

Since crisis intervention relies heavily on trained volunteers rather than licensed professionals, some approaches are designed for easy memorization and recall. For example, the SAFER-R model by George Everly:[3]

Stabilize
Acknowledge the crisis
Facilitate understanding
Encourage effective coping
Recovery or **R**eferral

Peggy Hartshorn offers a mnemonic-based pathway specifically suited to pregnancy crisis intervention called "The LOVE Approach."[4] Hartshorn describes the intervention process as follows:

Listen and Learn
Open Options
Vision and Value
Extend and Empower

While all of these suggested pathways are useful, the pathway presented below attempts to outline seven phases of pregnancy crisis intervention in the order most commonly experienced when you meet together. We will look at what to do and say in each phase.

Phase One: Listen and Assure

Assure her that you are there to help. Use her name often. Ask lots of questions. Listen to learn who she is and why being pregnant at this time is so upsetting for her. Sympathize with her worries and fears. Acknowledge the prime emotions: the embarrassment, the anger, and sense of abandonment or rejection. Mentally note what she says about her beliefs and feelings about her unborn child and the nature of her relationship with the father of her baby and her immediate family. You will circle back to these relationships later on.

In phase one, you are getting to know her and the precipitating events of her crisis. You're learning the names of the people involved, what they said, what she said, and what she thinks it all means now. You're assessing her personality and self-image. You're picking up her family history that has contributed to who she is now. You're noting her level of maturity and that of her partner. You're beginning to understand the dysfunction and brokenness among these key relationships. You're acknowledging that you understand the essential parts of her story as she shares them, and throughout, you're communicating your concern for her well-being.

In turn, she's relaxing a bit as she grows comfortable with you and can see that you care about her life. Forming this bond, or creating a sense of connection, is far less important in other forms of crisis counseling, but it's extremely foundational and necessary in pregnancy crisis intervention. Why?

Because pregnancy is about connectedness. As Frederica Mathewes-Green observes:

> Pregnancy is the icon of human intimacy. . . . When pregnancy begins, a woman is plunged into an experience of intimacy more profound than any of her adult life; she is knit, literally, to another human being, one half-made of her own self. In the same blow, she is linked to the child's father, whose half-life lives on in her body. Yet this being formed of two halves is more than their sum, a radical third never before seen on earth. . . .
>
> Pregnancy is about connectedness. It spins the wheel tighter and centrifugal force draws the players together, more aware than ever of their mutual dependence. *Pregnancy problems have to do with broken connections: broken trust, fear, loneliness, abandonment.*[5]

Helping a woman in a pregnancy-related crisis is largely the work of connecting and, where a relationship is broken, reconnecting. Mathewes-Green explains,

> There are many practical problems that must be solved in the course of an unplanned pregnancy. But the primary need appears to be to forge connections to other people, people that she can lean on through the difficult months ahead. This cannot be a superficial or faceless support. Women in listening groups frequently would say, "If I'd only had someone I could count on to stand by me," insisting that they meant someone really dependable, someone

who would care for them personally and who wouldn't let them down.[6]

In the initial phase of PCI counseling, what you are signaling is a readiness to be that someone. "Whatever happens, I will walk with you through this crisis." She is connecting with you. That is a good start.

Voices from the Field

Phase One: Listen
"Grandma Taught Me to Listen"

The first thing most people want is for someone just to listen to them. I learned this from my Grandma Alice. When I was in high school, any time I had something stressful in my life, I walked to her house and just hung out with her for a while. I don't remember her ever giving advice, but she always listened, she never judged, and it always helped.

In *Listening: The Forgotten Skill,* author Madelyn Burley-Allen says that when we listen from the heart, without judging, the speaker can experience emotional release and reduction of stress and tension. You will see this right away. Listening allows the woman in crisis to open up and share her concerns. This in turn helps you learn more about what resources may be helpful.

—Martha Shuping, MD

Phase Two: Identify and Amplify Her Values

Ask questions about her beliefs and values. Ask questions about her self-image. What kind of person does she see herself to be: independent, timid, determined, compassionate, uncertain, and so on. Ask, "How did you feel about abortion prior to this time? How did you come to form these views?" If she's already had an abortion, ask her about the antecedents and what happened afterwards. Listen keenly for the voice of ambivalence. Then slow down and help her hear it herself.

In phase two, you are looking to identify *her* heart values. In this sense, you truly are the pro-woman voice in her life. You want to help her make decisions based on those values rather than what is pragmatically easier, or pleasing, or what protects others.

Moral values are what make people strong. They go straight to a person's emotional well-being, self-esteem, and general outlook on life. Compromising those values leads to depression, self-loathing, and future self-destructive behavior.

In crisis, the person is not thinking clearly about her values. She wants quick relief—yielding to the pressures of others and rationalizing away what she really thinks is the quickest way to get relief. But the trauma that women experience after abortion starts right here, with not listening to their own hearts and consciences and finding the strength within themselves to follow that path. Cathi Butwell writes:

> [The abortion clinic counselor] said to me, "I know you're feeling bad. But when I had an abortion, my kids asked me if that wasn't killing a baby. And I told them that if you step on an acorn, that's not killing an oak tree. It's just a seed. It's O.K. to kill a seed." So instead of following my own conscience, which was telling me to get out of there, I sat there trying real hard to hang on to that and tried to believe that the baby wasn't alive. . . . But I was sick to my stomach for days. I had finally realized what I had done. It was all I could think about. I had just killed my baby. Nobody could ever accept me if they knew.[7]

Yielding and rationalizing like this leads to depression and self-loathing. In Cathi's case, she expresses it in her conclusion, "Nobody could ever accept me if they knew."

This is the time in the crisis intervention process to slow down women like Cathi and help them think through their beliefs and values (religious or not). Abortion clearly solves some problems and produces others. Help her anticipate how surrendering her values to others or rationalizing them away will affect her afterward.

You've already learned why she thinks she needs an abortion. Now ask, "What is it about abortion you don't believe in?" She may take a roundabout way of expressing the answer. Be patient and help her get there.

> She may say blankly, "I just don't like it."
> You ask, "What is it about abortion that you don't like?"
> "It's wrong," she may offer.
> "Why is it wrong?"
> She may answer, "It's against my religion" (or she may just repeat herself).
> "What is your religion, and what does it teach you?"
> "I'm a Baptist, and they say abortion is wrong."
> "Why do Baptists teach abortion is wrong?"
> "They say it's killing."
> "What is it killing?"
> "It's taking a life."
> "What life?"
> "The life of a baby."

There's her heart! Now clarify and amplify *her* heart values:

> So what you're telling me is that in spite of all the difficult circumstances you've told me about, and in spite of the strong temptation to solve your problems through abortion, you believe abortion is wrong. It's wrong because it's intentionally killing an innocent human being. And you don't see yourself as the kind of person who would ever hurt an innocent child. I can see why you might be relieved on one hand but devastated on the other. Am I hearing you correctly?

Now she understands her own ambivalence. She's clarified her own values. She has spoken aloud to you and to herself what she honestly believes abortion is but has been afraid to say or unable to articulate until now. She has separated out what she really wants from what she is supposed to want (according to our cultural leaders).

In phase two, you're helping the woman in pregnancy distress identify and amplify her own values. You've said nothing about what you believe or value. You're exploring her heart. You're not focused at this moment on the unborn child's well-being but on the woman's health and well-being, relative to her unborn child. They are connected. Her own moral or religious values, her sense of self-esteem and self-image, her own sense of inner strength and pride, her ability to think about short-term versus long-term consequences—any of these may be the avenue that allows her to see what is truly best.

In summary, phase two involves a major reconnection. You're helping her reconnect with herself: "What do I really believe, and how then should I live?" Can she envision her religious or moral beliefs now to be a source of guidance and strength to overcome the crisis in a life-affirming way? Can she see how giving birth and making a parenting plan may be harder but will make her proud of herself and leave no lasting regret? If she believes in God, how will aborting affect that relationship? If she's not religious, ask it in a nonreligious way. "How do you think violating your own conscience will change you? How will yielding to the beliefs and demands of others affect those relationships?"

At this point, a major transition occurs. You transition from asking, listening, and mirroring to educating and confirming information relative to her pregnancy.

Phase Three: Confirm and Inform Her Options

Using fetal models and science brochures and, if possible, ultrasound provide medically accurate information on fetal development, miscarriage, and birth. Using fact sheets or other medical resources, educate her about abortion procedures and health risks. Provide answers to FAQs about parenting help, adoption, maternity homes, and so on as appropriate.

If she has expressed ambivalence about abortion and clarified why, then phase three allows you to confirm her values using science. If she has expressed no ambivalence, phase three is more educational, a matter of informed consent about her intentions. In phase three you are confirming, correcting, and educating people about pregnancy, fetal development and pregnancy outcomes.

In a PHO setting, phase three is typically when a pregnancy test is provided, and if the test is positive, then a confirmation of pregnancy is done through ultrasound. A positive pregnancy test usually, but not always, means that she is pregnant.[8] It can never confirm viability. Standard of care within the medical field requires ultrasound verification of an intact uterine pregnancy prior to giving a pregnancy diagnosis, something only a licensed medical professional can do. You can, however, discuss the test procedure and talk about the results and why ultrasound confirmation is important before making any decisions about outcomes.

For those women intending to undergo a surgical abortion, ultrasound verification is medically indicated for its own reasons. First, surgical abortion is medically unnecessary if ultrasound indicates a miscarriage. Second, ultrasound is used to determine gestational age. Gestational age indicates the type of abortion procedure required and the physical risks associated with it. Few women intending abortion for the first time have a factual understanding of procedures and risks.

Nor do they have a clear understanding of fetal science. Fetal models, fetal science brochures, and ultrasound serve to confirm why being pregnant is commonly expressed as "having a baby." Even more, you're helping her understand *her* pregnancy.

If phase one involves the young woman connecting with you as a dependable friend in the midst of her crisis, and phase two is about reconnecting her with her own values and sense of self, then phase three brings us to a third connection point: connecting the mother, or couple, with their own unborn child.[9]

Next, there are outcomes to discuss: miscarriage, abortion, and birth. Studies of miscarriage rates vary widely, from 5 to 70 percent depending on what factors are considered. But for our purposes, we may affirm that for women who know they are pregnant, the risk of miscarriage before twenty weeks is between 8 and 20 percent.[10]

For this reason, ultrasound verification of a viable pregnancy is important. A percentage will discover that they don't have a viable pregnancy. Ultrasound may confirm the absence of a heartbeat, indicating a fetal demise. Or there may be an unusually high or low heart rate, indicating a possible impending miscarriage.[11] In such cases, waiting a week or two and then returning for a repeat ultrasound is advised.

If the woman is considering abortion, then this is the time to explain the procedures and risks. For example, the nonsurgical abortion option, typically called the Abortion Pill (RU-486), by its very name leaves the impression that the process is a single-dose procedure. In reality, the Food and Drug Administration explains that this procedure is designed to involve several pills and multiple office visits.[12]

The FDA-approved procedure involves three visits. During the first visit, RU-486 pill(s) are given. This pill blocks pregnancy hormones that support the embryo. Two days later, during a second visit, the woman returns for the second medication, which will cause the uterus to cramp and expel the pregnancy. A few weeks later, a third visit is required to confirm that the abortion is complete. If the abortion is incomplete, (which occurs five to eight times out of a hundred cases), RU-486 may be given again or a first-trimester surgical abortion procedure may be done. This is the procedure upon which the FDA approved the use of the abortion pill.

In practice, however, "many clinics give both sets of pills at the first visit and eliminate the second visit. So, the woman is most commonly at home with no medical supervision when the cramping and bleeding begin."[13]

Surgical abortion procedures change depending on gestational age. The physical risks increase with gestational age. At this moment in your conversation with her, now is the time to use medically accurate brochures or resources to explain abortion procedures and risks.

Finally, there is the birth option followed by a decision to parent or place the baby for adoption. You have plenty of time to work out the parenting or adoption plans once she has decided to give birth. For many, phase three results in women expressing a desire to have her baby but uncertain about it due to her difficult circumstances. This is your signal that another transition is occurring.

VOICES FROM THE FIELD

Phase Three: Confirm Options
"The Adoption Option"

Macy was a track star in high school. She earned a scholarship and would be the first one in her family to go to college. When Macy got pregnant, her first thought was abortion. She had her whole life ahead of her. Macy's boyfriend, however, begged her not to abort. He promised to help her raise the baby, but he was also going away to college on a full scholarship. Parenting seemed impossible. Abortion seemed wrong.

We talked with her about how she could be a part of this baby's life and still go forward with her own life plans. We introduced the open adoption option. Then we took her into the ultrasound room. The ultrasound revealed a lively baby girl, already twenty-four weeks along. That's when her heart was changed against abortion. In the days that followed, we met with Macy's mother and everyone came together around an open adoption plan. Macy and her boyfriend are no longer together, but they are still part of little Bella's life through pictures and holiday visits.

—Martha Avila, Heartbeat of Miami

Phase Four: Direct and Appeal

You've communicated your love for her and your concern for her future. You've taken the time to slow things down and ask questions that get to the heart of the matter. You've provided accurate medical information regarding pregnancy and its outcomes. Now you're looking to understand how the information provided is affecting her thinking.

On her side of the counseling experience, she's connected with you and feels less alone. She's reconnected with her own values and sense of self. And hopefully, she's starting to connect with her unborn child.

Abortion once seemed like the perfect solution. The petals have fallen off that rose, and the thorns have shown themselves. Emotionally, she is back to the starting point and asks, "What should I do?" She's asking you for direction.

The skillful counselor will provide decision-making guidance by asking, "Have you considered…" or, "What if you did such and such…" and then giving her a suggested pathway. It's not unusual to hear, "I really want to have my baby," while the tone conveys a longing, not a resolution. In this case, she needs direction in the sense of simple encouragement. "Do it then. It's okay."

Remember Norm Wright's advice: "In crisis counseling, the person . . . must see that they need to make a choice to remain the same or to change and grow. . . . A goal of crisis counseling is to help the person in need accept and take responsibility."[14] Then the hard work of moving forward can begin.

What you're really saying is, "Have faith. Things will work out." If she has already indicated that she believes in God, openly return to her own faith. Ask if this is not a time to call upon him, follow his will, and trust him to provide. For many women and couples, this represents still another reconnecting point: returning to the God they believe in and calling on him for help.

But if this seems uncomfortable for either of you, keep it more personal. For example, "Follow your heart." Or, "Be true to your own values."

Or you may broaden out the appeal still further. Remind her of the common human experience: that our hardest challenges often turn out to be the proudest and most satisfying accomplishments of our lives. That is the narrative of many mothers in difficult circumstances amid an unplanned pregnancy. A young mom resolves to give life to her baby and then finds a way to do so, even at great personal sacrifice. Looking back, she sees it as one of her greatest achievements.

In this phase, you're encouraging her to make a firm decision. On occasion, this may also mean warning or cautioning her about unwanted outcomes. For example, she may say, "I know it's not right. But I'm going to get an abortion. It's the only way my boyfriend won't leave me. I can't lose him."

You might express the caution, "None of us want to be alone. But I would caution you to think that choice and outcome through. Many women who abort to please and keep a man end up hating him and losing him soon after. These women report a profound sense of loss and regret."

As long as you speak respectfully, you can direct, appeal, and warn her in wholly appropriate ways. Don't be afraid to do so. This is part of speaking the truth in love.

Phase Five: Problem-Solve and Plan

If she expresses a desire to give life in spite of her difficulties, turn immediately to problem-solving and planning. Circle back to each of the main characters in her story and discuss communicating her desire to each one. Make suggestions that directly and specifically solve immediate problems.

For example, you may ask, "How would you like to tell your parents?" You could suggest, "Would you like me to be with you?" Or perhaps: "Let's consider their response and prepare for it." Or you could ask, "You told me that your boyfriend would support you, whatever you decided. Do you think he will truly support your decision, which will make him a father? Should we bring him in to see the ultrasound and go through the reasons why you now want to have your baby?"

In this phase, you are problem-solving and making implementation plans. Nothing in her particular circumstances has been altered in any way. She's just had time to reconnect with her own values and self-image. She's had the opportunity to connect with her unborn child. She's no longer feeling the despair of being alone. She's not as afraid, and she's a little more hopeful.

She doesn't know what she will do in terms of raising the baby, getting married, continuing or suspending her education, placing for adoption, or finding the finances needed for what she ultimately arranges. She only knows what she will not do now: she will not abort her baby.

However, do not assume the crisis is over. Monitoring is still important because the pressure of others, including threats and direct actions designed to force her into an abortion, can occur. Anticipating this possibility, you will help her make a plan for standing by her decision before the end of your time together.

At this point, your focus is not on answering the big questions that make up the final resolution. That will come in time. The focus is on planning how best to communicate her life-affirming decision to the people in her social network so they will eventually affirm her decision and support it. The focus here once again is on reconnection.

If she anticipates anger, threats, or violence, then you need to find out what preparations need to be made before she tells them. For example, if she expects to be kicked out of her home as a way of compelling her to have an abortion, then you need to discuss with her where she can go that is safe and supportive. Often such a place is needed only for a week or two, until emotions calm down and her decision to stand for life is irrefutably demonstrated. After this, most of the time, people relent and begin to show support. But this is not always the case and a maternity home may be needed long term.

She may now desperately want to have her baby but equally feel unable to do it without the support of her partner or family. She may say, "If they support me, I know I could do it."

Then plan for the next step only. Suggest, "Okay, let's not make any final decisions right now. But let's plan for you to return tomorrow with your partner (or parent/s) and go through the process again with them. Let them see your heart's desire and why."

Phase Six: Empower and Promise

Provide her with some take-home materials to review or to use for explaining her decision to others. Schedule a follow-up. Give her your phone number. Get her phone number. Pray with her if appropriate. Promise to help her over the coming weeks and months. Be specific when possible. For example, plan together what she is going to do over the next 24 to 48 hours. Who will she talk to? When? Where? As you bring your time together to a close, reassure her of your long-term support and prepare her to return to her disordered world.

If her intention to abort remains unchanged, you may express some final concerns. "It saddens me to see you go that way. If at any point you change your mind, please call me. My offer to help you find an alternative still stands."

Otherwise, offer final words of encouragement. Speak to her inner strength and moral courage. "If you stand up for your unborn child and patiently endure all the shouting and threats, you can, and will, win this battle. Can you find it within yourself to do this?"

Many can, when encouraged to do so. As the psalmist testified, "For by you I can run against a troop, and by my God I can leap over a wall" (18:29).

101

Phase Seven: Monitor and Mentor

Keep in touch. Keep it personal. Monitor the reaction of her partner or parents, and monitor her reaction to them. Make sure she starts prenatal care. Help her create a parenting plan over the subsequent weeks and months.

In this follow-up phase, which can be days to months long, you will be monitoring the ongoing crisis. You will make sure she reconnects with her partner, family, and community of friends, as appropriate, around her decision to give birth. When this is not possible, then you can introduce her to a substitute support system, such as a safe home for mothers, a small group from the PHO, or an adoption agency.

The critical factor to monitor is the secrecy of the pregnancy itself. No matter how much a young mother says that she wants to have her baby, as long as her pregnancy remains a secret, she is at risk for abortion. This means the crisis is ongoing and monitoring is required.

You are also mentoring her toward a parenting plan. She may parent the child herself or select parents for her child. She may get married as part of that plan or work out child support and visitation. She may want to take classes to prepare to be a mom. Her partner may want to learn about fatherhood.

Remember, pregnancy crisis is about disconnection. Pregnancy crisis intervention is the process of reconnection.

7

EFFECTIVE CRISIS INTERVENTION SKILLS

"I will never forget what you said. Thank you. It changed my life."

—Arianna

"A word fitly spoken is like apples of gold in a setting of silver."

—Proverbs 25:11

Women and couples in pregnancy distress present their crisis verbally and nonverbally, in part and haphazardly, with distorted perspective and bits of misinformation. They may show joy and fear along with anger and hope in alternating waves of expression. They feel out of control and may think they are going crazy. But since the event is real and life-altering, their sense of crisis is rational.

You're trying to take it all in, sort fact from fiction, understand motives and intentions, assess the depth of their crisis, and clarify in your mind the initial steps of an intervention plan. To help you in this process, there are basic counseling tools at your disposal. These tools, or skills, are naturally yours in some degree. With some forethought and intentionality on your part, you can improve these skills and with them, your effectiveness as a counselor. Professional training in crisis intervention counseling begins with *basic* counseling skills. I will introduce these skills in the context of pregnancy crisis intervention.

1. Micro-Messaging

In the beginning, we emphasized that if you love people—specifically, if you genuinely care for people in a pregnancy-related crisis—then you can do an adequate job of pregnancy crisis intervention without formal training. That's because love is a powerful guide. It especially controls what is commonly called "micro-messaging." These are the messages you send without much thinking (or training). These are the messages you emote by your level of eye contact, facial expressions, body position, touch, and tone of voice.

How effective are these nonverbal messages in establishing a working relationship? Sheila Jackson-Cherry and Bradley Erford report,

> In one study, R.P. Bedi surveyed clients who had received counseling and asked them to identify the specific counselor behaviors that most helped to form a working alliance. Following validation and education, clients ranked nonverbal gestures and presentation and body language as the most important alliance-building factors. These nonverbal attending behaviors communicate a counselor's interest, warmth, and understanding to the client and include behaviors such as eye contact, body position, and tone of voice.[1]

If the controlling emotion of your life in the midst of counseling is frustration or anger, it will be reflected in your body language and facial expressions. The woman or couple will detect an unspoken condemnation of their choices or a feeling of being judged. Minimally, they will sense that you are peeved or put out by their presence and the demands they are making on your time. Obviously, this will affect their response to you and everything that follows.

On the other hand, if the dominant emotion of your life in the intervention process is loving concern, the frightened and anxious young woman will detect it immediately through multiple micro-messages. Your smile, your tone of voice, and more will welcome her. It will lower her fears and start the relationship needed to work through the complex issues creating the crisis. Whatever limitations you have in medical knowledge and counseling experience are more likely to be overlooked. She likes you because you genuinely care for her. That's a start.

Effective and experienced counselors are aware of the micro-messages they send and become quite intentional about sending them. These include eye contact, body position, vocal tone, touch, and silence, as described in more detail below.

Eye contact: In some African and Asian cultures, eye contact is how the authority-subordinate relationship is acknowledged. The one in authority uses eye contact; the subordinate does not. In such contexts, strong eye contact may imply defiance or disrespect. But in American and European culture, maintaining strong eye contact signals keen interest and attentiveness. It shows that your focus is on her and not elsewhere. Good eye contact is not a stare down. It naturally breaks off and then resets. Focused eyes send the message that you care about her well-being and are concerned about her state of upheaval. This immediately lowers anxiety and signals permission for her to tell you her story.

Therefore, maintain good eye contact if you want her to know you are "all in" when it comes to her crisis. You may be curious about what time it is, but looking at a clock or at your watch is a serious error. Keep your phone off and out of sight. A little self-control concerning eye contact will keep you on message.

Note, however, that in the context of PCI, the woman may not look back. She may stare at the floor or focus on your hands or her own. Her avoidance is usually an expression of shame and embarrassment. In such cases, let her be. As she sees you are not there to pass judgment, she will begin to connect with you, eye to eye.

Body position: Generally, sitting close indicates care and sitting at a distance indicates emotional distance. Sitting behind a desk is certain to cut off any sense that she has found a safe harbor to disclose her secret anguish.

Body distance and position should reflect both your respect for her as an autonomous human being and your concern for her as a person in crisis. Sit far enough away so she doesn't feel you are encroaching on her. But sit close enough to hand her a tissue with ease or to look over a brochure together. Sit in a way so you can speak face to face. Sit with an open and calm demeanor, and avoid crossing your arms.

Vocal Tone: "The pitch, pacing and volume can all have an effect on how a client responds emotionally to a crisis counselor."[2] We are all familiar with the objection, "It's not what you said but how you said it!" Tone conveys the heart. A soft tone using a controlled pace signals a sympathetic readiness to hear of her plight. This is the starting point. A more normal tone and a professional manner are good when you are informing her about a pregnancy test, fetal development, and pregnancy or abortion procedures and risks. Near the end, your pitch may rise slightly as you seek to encourage her in the steps she is taking.

Touch: Touch signals different messages in different cultures. It's necessary to understand this. In the West, a female counselor can guide a young woman to a seat using touch. A female counselor may pat or even hold her hand reassuringly at certain points when she is struggling to express herself.

Male counselors must be much more restrained. My advice is to refrain from any touch until the end of your time together, unless you are talking to your daughter or sister or another person with whom you have a close relationship.

Just as there are male and female OBGYN doctors, there are also male and female crisis counselors. Men in each case must be aware of the male-female dynamic and adjust accordingly. In our current context, men should not convey their concern by touch but instead through a respectful, serious demeanor. When wrapping up, when her trust is high, a handshake will convey a professional compassion she will appreciate. Remember, pregnancy crisis, by definition, involves a man. More often than not, she is feeling hurt or disappointed by him. Often (but *not* always), he is a self-centered and immature male. For this reason, most pregnancy help clinics primarily train women for PCI counseling. Mature men can and do make a powerful contribution in this setting, but they must adjust. In my case, these adjustments meant counseling primarily with couples that come in or meeting with the male partner separately. In cases where I have sat down with a young woman in a pregnancy-related crisis, I have a female PCI counselor-in-training with me. Others may decide differently, and in other cultures, the norms may be different. But these are worth considering.

Silence: Used in small and timely measures, silence is an effective tool in conveying patience. If you are nervous, you will tend to talk. Control this nervousness with silence. But keep in mind that if the silence is too long, it may generate anxiety in her.

Silence is also an effective tool to use when your discussion reaches a moment of decision. To regain control of her life and take responsibility for what follows, she alone must make the decision. It's up to her to speak to her boyfriend or parents or to make a critical call. Silence signals the importance of the moment and the need for her to determine her next steps.

2. Intentional Listening

Listening is another valuable basic skill in pregnancy crisis intervention. Listening is far more than hearing. By intentional listening, I mean active, focused, intensified listening. Good listeners are people who sit down with someone and intentionally set aside their "to do" list. You may have many demands on your time. But for now, the woman or couple in pregnancy crisis is the priority. Close out the voices of others in the hallway, traffic noises, alerts on your phone. As you listen, don't think about how to respond or react with words or facial expressions.

Intentional listening is a gathering and receiving tool. It's what you use to get to know her—to understand her situation, her feelings, the key players in her life, her deepest desires/values, as well as the pressure points that are driving the crisis at that moment. Being a good listener usually requires you to start with clarifying questions. Ask and listen. Ask and listen.

3. Clarifying Questions

In the context of pregnancy crisis intervention, there are about a dozen clarifying questions you can use to guide you as a beginner in PCI counseling (which are provided in Appendix 1). These are a combination of open and closed questions.

Closed questions: Closed questions are yes and no questions or questions that can be answered in a few words. Closed questions establish facts. In the context of PCI, such questions may include: How old are you? Have you had a pregnancy test? Have you been pregnant before? What was the outcome? Are you married or unmarried? What was the first day of your last menstrual period (LMP)? Are you here alone or is someone with you?

These kinds of closed questions establish whether you are speaking to an adult or a minor, to someone who has had multiple and casual sexual relationships or is "in love" and pregnant for the first time. You learn whether you are talking to someone who fears she might be pregnant but may not be, or someone who shows multiple indications of pregnancy and knows how far along she is. If she has already had one, two, or three abortions, it helps you know what kind of open questions to ask. Closed questions quickly identify the people involved and her relationship to them.

PHOs typically use an intake form that allows you to ask and note closed questions regarding her medical and pregnancy history. By starting with a few closed questions, you provide her with time to relax; they are easy to answer and also help you establish a calm, professional demeanor.

Open questions: Open questions bring us to the heart of the matter. They are the questions that reveal stories and beliefs, feelings and hopes. For example, ask "What fears do you have about being pregnant at this time?" and then listen. Open questions are used to understand the events that led to the crisis. Why is this pregnancy a crisis? Open questions explain the nature or quality of her relationship with the man in her life. "Can you tell me about your current relationship? Does he see your relationship in the same way or differently? How do you know?" Asking open questions is the main tool you use to understand who she is, her level of understanding, the amount of coercion or autonomy she is experiencing, and so on.

VOICES FROM THE FIELD

Clarifying Questions
"Ask Clarifying Questions"

In a recent phone conversation, a young woman said, "I think I need an abortion." After explaining that we don't perform or refer for abortions, I homed in on her word *think.* I asked, "Why do you *think* you need one?" She felt she couldn't afford another baby. I asked her what her understanding of abortion was. She replied that it was "killing a baby." But two friends told her she needed to do what was right for her and not to think about the baby.

I then asked if she knew anyone who had had an abortion. It turned out that the very two friends who were encouraging her to abort had both aborted. I asked her what they said about their experience. She said they both regretted their decision. I summarized, "So, your friends who regret aborting their babies are telling you to abort yours?" She hesitated, then replied with a shaky "yes" and began crying. She ended our conversation with "I'm so glad I called. I needed to hear what you had to say." A few days later she confirmed that she would carry to term.

—Wendy Merrill, First Choice Pregnancy Center

4. Mirroring and Paraphrasing

Mirroring is simply restating the woman's views or feelings as she expresses them, but in your own words. Paraphrasing is similar in that it allows you to summarize what she has told you over the last several minutes. Counselors use mirroring and paraphrasing for two reasons. First, it's a tool for cross-checking that you are hearing accurately what she is telling you (or revealing anything that you have misunderstood). Second, mirroring and paraphrasing allows her to clarify her own thoughts and feelings. You are not repeating her words; you are recasting them.

Why is this helpful? Remember, crisis makes it hard for a person to think clearly. Therefore, in crisis counseling, mirroring and paraphrasing are especially helpful in that they bring clarity to both you and the woman in the pregnancy crisis. Hearing you say what she has just tried to say is often helpful when she's had a hard time thinking and expressing herself. Realizing that another person genuinely understands her conflicting feelings and desires is also a tension-releasing moment for her.

For example, I might ask an open question such as, "How did you feel about abortion prior to this current crisis?" This question cuts through the immediate pressures of her situation and allows her to express something of her life values and belief system (moral/religious).

A common response is, "I never thought I would have one." This is a revealing moment for her. She is now hearing her own words, expressing something deep inside of her.

If I ask her why she never wanted or expected an abortion for herself, she will most likely tell me that abortion is a negative thing in her mind. She may even express something of the humanity of the unborn child. "I know it's wrong." Or even more directly, "It kills a baby."

Most women considering abortion will express deep reservations if asked. Women struggling with abortion grief are often most regretful that they did not listen to themselves or have the power to stand up for what they truly wanted. The key people in her life dismissed her reservations or suppressed her own thoughts and values. But afterward, those people moved on and she was left alone, wrestling with those same values and how abortion changed her. Mirroring is the tool to use for amplifying her own voice of conscience before the outcome is decided.

Mirroring her here, I might say, "Am I correct that you are saying that in spite of this current difficult situation, and the fear of possibly being alone, you believe abortion is wrong or a bad thing to do?"

If she responds with "Yes, that's right," then I know I have understood her. More important, she has heard from her own mouth to her own ears, echoed and amplified by me, her true belief system.

Our discussion might well have gone into her church or religious background, how she was taught as a child, or how she always viewed herself. Paraphrasing this important moment, I might say, "So are you telling me that you believe abortion is wrong because it kills a baby and you are only considering it now because of the painful circumstance you are in?"

If she agrees, you have now helped her see the value of looking at all other options before doing what she in truth does not want to do.

5. Accurately Communicating

While you don't need to be an expert in pregnancy health issues, you do need to communicate accurate medical information about pregnancy, fetal development, abortion procedures and risks, miscarriage rates, and prenatal care.

If you are preparing to do pregnancy crisis intervention through your local pregnancy help clinic, your training will include a review of medically accurate information. In the PCI counselor's toolkit, basic medical knowledge regarding pregnancy (menstrual cycle, LMP versus gestational age, fetal development, abortion procedures, and so on) is one of the most effective and commonly used tools.

Learn the material and become familiar with the brochures or apps used to provide women or couples with the information they need as part of "informed consent." Gain a level of comfort in sharing the medical information simply and in ways she can adapt should she want to share the materials with others in her circle of support. Knowledge of this material, and the ability to talk about it accurately and clearly, is essential for PCI counselors.

6. Decision-Making Guidance

Don't tell her what to do. Counseling by its very nature avoids giving direct advice: "Here's what I think you ought to do…" In the context of PCI, remember that people have been telling her what to do for weeks. She doesn't need more of the same. Instead, give her the space to think on her own and to make her own decisions. You can still provide decision-making guidance. After all, if she had felt capable of making decisions without any guidance, she would not have turned to you.

The skillful counselor will provide decision-making guidance by asking, "Have you considered…" or "What if you did such and such…" In this way, you are treating her as an adult who is responsible for the outcome of this crisis. She may have been victimized along the way, but you will not treat her as a victim going forward. Victims have no sense of control or responsibility. In fact, unless she is a minor, she is responsible for the pregnancy outcome. Even as a minor, with parental or guardian involvement, she has patient rights regarding her pregnancy and medical treatment.

At times, a woman may plead with you, "Please tell me what to do!" In those situations, I've offered short counsel that still requires them to own their decision and to take responsibility for all that follows from it. I've said, "I would encourage you to follow your heart." Or, I might say, "It looks like you have to decide between doing what is right and doing what is easy." I've offered, "If you decide to have this baby, in spite of all the difficulties of your current situation, I will be here to help you. But this is a decision you have to make and live with."

7. Tender Confrontation

In the field of crisis intervention, professional training guidelines provide for such times when a counselor must respectfully and tenderly confront the person in crisis. In these situations, there is a deep discrepancy between a person's expected outcome and what, in reality, will most likely happen.

The clearest example I can provide is in the context of a suicide. Say someone tells you, "I'm going to jump off this bridge. Everybody will be a lot happier if I am just out of the picture." You cannot respond, "I want you to know, I really care about you and will support your decision either way." No, some decisions are reckless, unlawful, and destructive. Failure to confront in such a moment is usually rooted not in what is best for her but in not wanting to be rejected or criticized.

It is not uncommon for a woman in pregnancy crisis to say, "I know abortion is terribly wrong. It's really against my beliefs. But it's the only way out of my situation." Responding with tender confrontation, you might say, "I am sorry to hear that. Abortion does solve problems. But I caution you, from a mental health perspective, that doing what you believe is terribly wrong and aborting your own values creates traumatic new problems I want to spare you from if possible." Or you might say, "I'm sorry you think that. But before you do what you believe is terribly wrong, please consider the experience of others who felt the same prior to their abortion. Not all but many women report months, even years, of emotional pain. Depression, guilt, grieving, and self-destructive behaviors are strongly associated with abortion. If you change your mind, I am here to help you find a life-affirming solution. Please feel free to return."

Tender confrontation is also needed when a woman is being defrauded into abortion. A man sat with me as his girlfriend spoke with our female PCI counselor. He said to me, "She needs to have an abortion. The truth is, things are not good. I'm planning on breaking up with her."

"Does she know that?" I asked him. "Is she considering abortion to please you, in order to keep your relationship going?" She was. In this case, he was the one who needed confrontation. "Either we go in together with her and you tell her honestly what she can expect from you as she makes this life or death decision, or I will tell her."

Be on the alert for these commonly expressed relationship-related reluctant abortions. Here the woman is resorting to abortion because she expects it will secure her ongoing relationship. A typical expression might be: "My boyfriend says he is absolutely not ready to be a father. He insists that I have an abortion or he will leave me. I need him so much."

Part of the gnawing anguish of abortion grief comes from this very scenario. The woman aborts to please her partner and soon after resents him so much that she ends the relationship. Michaelene's narrative of her abortion experience (provided in chapter 4) was an example of this sad but common reality. It was her boyfriend who insisted on abortion if their relationship was to continue. She pleaded for him to look at alternatives but to no avail. After relenting to him, she writes, "The mere presence of my boyfriend caused deep hurt and pain. . . . Desperate for a fresh start, I broke up with my boyfriend."[3]

This dynamic works in the opposite direction as well. Zach writes,

When my girlfriend told me she was pregnant, I knew the baby was mine; I knew I'd take care of it. I loved her. I wanted to marry her. I would have raised the child alone, if that's what she wanted. She said she was having an abortion and that was it. I didn't feel good about it, but I was determined to support her decision. I wanted our relationship to last. But we were both changed afterward. I tried to keep us together but things kept getting worse until we finally broke it off.[4]

Aborting an unborn child against your own heartfelt values is not a bonding experience. It tears you apart.

Tender confrontation is the art of pointing out discrepancies between decisions made and expected outcomes. Tender confrontation means willingness to challenge a false assumption. But be sure to always do it in love.

VOICES FROM THE FIELD

Tenderly Confronting
"Young Man, Speak Up!"

Men are taught that they're not allowed to speak their mind about abortion and that it's just her decision. I've often heard guys say to their girlfriends, "I'll be there for you no matter what you choose." They are doing their best to be supportive, but they don't think they can actually say, "I want to have our baby. We can do this." What she *hears* in the "I'll support your decision either way" statement is that he won't even be there to help her make a decision. It makes her feel abandoned and more alone. So, when you hear a man talk like this, tease out want he really is saying. She needs to hear him loud and clear say, "I want our baby to live. You are not alone. We can do this together."

—Melinda Gardner, Apple Pregnancy Care Center

8. Encouraging

Encouragement is not about saying complimentary things. It's about strengthening weak knees. It's helping people see that they have more power than they sense in the moment. Encouragement is the skill of helping people see themselves at their best and act accordingly.

Encouragement is not "Pollyannaish" or a positive thinking exercise. You do well to acknowledge hard realities. But the truly balanced perspective acknowledges another reality: Our proudest achievements in life are almost always grounded in doing what is hard and overcoming great difficulties. That reminder is what we mean by encouragement.

Encouragement says, "Yes it's hard, but you can do it. You can have your baby and graduate from college. Of course, it's harder to accomplish with a baby on your knee. But you will not be the first to accomplish it. It can be done."

Encouragement is realistic and empowering. It says, "You probably will need help from family and friends. It will probably take an extra year to finish, maybe more. But when you walk across that stage to receive your diploma, knowing all that it took to accomplish, you will be proud of yourself."

Proverbs 25:11 says, "A word fitly spoken is like apples of gold in a setting of silver." Often this "apple of gold" is a fitly spoken word of encouragement when it matters most.

Concluding Thoughts

Pregnancy is a normal, common, everyday experience, like marriage or even death. But when someone you love dies, it's a dramatic event for you and can be a traumatic experience. In the same way, pregnancy is one of the most singularly meaningful events in all human experience. Commonly, it's a welcome and fulfilling experience. But just as commonly, it's a crisis.

Thank you for providing life-affirming help at such a time. It's one of the finest things you will ever do. If the outcome is abortion, nonetheless, you were a witness to the truth and love of life. If it does work out well, then for years to come, indeed, for the rest of your life, your intervention will give you a sense of satisfaction—of being used in a meaningful way in the life of a mother and her child.

APPENDICES

Appendix 1

TWELVE QUESTIONS TO GUIDE BEGINNERS IN PCI

If you are anxious that you might say or do the wrong thing, then work through the following questions with the young woman or couple. This will be of great help to her.

1. How do you know you are pregnant? Have you had a hospital quality pregnancy test?

2. How far along are you? When was your last menstrual period?

3. Have you had an ultrasound verification that you have a viable pregnancy and are not about to miscarry?

4. Have you been pregnant before? What happened?

5. What fears do you have about being pregnant right now?

6. What is abortion? If your circumstances were different, what would you do? Why?

7. What do you know about fetal development? How developed is your unborn?

8. Since abortion is surgery, do you understand the procedures? The risks?

9. Is there anyone who would support your decision to give birth?

10. Tell me about your faith and values. What do they teach you to do? Do you believe there is a God who created your baby? Who cares about you? Would you like me to pray?

11. What would need to happen for you to give birth to your baby?

12. What is your phone number? I will stay with you through this crisis.

Appendix 2

PREGNANCY CRISIS INTERVENTION RESOURCES

Pregnancy Crisis Helpline

"Option Line" is a 24/7 (365 days a year) pregnancy helpline serving those in crisis pregnancy

Phone 1–800–712-HELP (4357), text "Helpline" to 313131, or visit the website at https://www.heartbeatinternational.org/ol-hb

Local Pregnancy Help Center Locator: Worldwide Directory

https://www.heartbeatinternational.org/worldwide-directory

Pregnancy Intervention Training and Support Organizations

Heartbeat International: www.heartbeatinternational.org

Care Net: www.care-net.org

National Institute for Family and Life Advocates: www.nifla.org

Embrace Grace: www.embracegrace.com

Legal Protection against Forced Abortion

Center against Forced Abortion, The Justice Foundation: http://thejusticefoundation.org/cafa/

Pregnancy Crisis Case Studies

Ford, Amy. *A Bump in Life: True Stories of Hope and Courage during an Unplanned Pregnancy.* Nashville: B & H Books, 2013.

Kuebelbeck, Amy, and Deborah L. Davis. *A Gift of Time: Continuing Your Pregnancy When Your Baby's Life Is Expected to Be Brief.* Baltimore, MD: The Johns Hopkins University Press, 2011.

After Abortion Grief

Abortion Changes You: www.abortionchangesyou.com

Abortion Recovery International: http://abortionrecovery.org

Appendix 3

"VOICES FROM THE FIELD" CONTRIBUTORS

Martha Avila
Heartbeat of Miami
Miami, Florida

Peggy Benicke
Robbinsdale Women's Center
Minneapolis, Minnesota

Melinda Gardner
Apple Pregnancy Care Center
Eau Claire, Wisconsin

Wendy Merrill
First Choice Pregnancy Center
Waterville, Maine

Vikki Parker
Option Pregnancy Center
Cabot, Arkansas

Jeanne Pernia
PassionLife
Miami, Florida

Martha Shuping, MD
Psychiatrist (private practice)
Winston-Salem, North Carolina

Tina Williams
Alpha Pregnancy Resource Center
Sanford, Maine

Notes

Introduction

1. On the worldwide incidence of abortion, see G. Sedgh, et al., "Abortion Incidence between 1990 and 2014: Global, Regional, and Sub-regional Levels and Trends, *The Lancet* (2016), http://www.thelancet.com/journals/lancet/article/PIIS0140-6736(16)30380-4/abstract.

2. The Guttmacher Institute Fact Sheet, "Global Incidence and Trends," https://www.guttmacher.org/fact-sheet/induced-abortion-worldwide.

3. Burl E. Gilliland and Richard K. James, *Crisis Intervention Strategies*, 8th ed. (Boston: Cengage Learning, 2016), 6 (emphasis added).

4. George S. Everly Jr., *Assisting Individuals in Crisis*, 5th ed. (Ellicott City, MD: International Critical Incident Foundation, 2015), 16.

Chapter 1

1. Heath Lambert, *A Theology of Biblical Counseling* (Grand Rapids: Zondervan, 2016), 13.

2. "Q and A with Bernard Nathanson," *Focus on the Family Citizen Magazine* (August 26, 1996), 7.

Chapter 2

1. Lisa R. Jackson-Cherry and Bradley T. Erford, *Crisis Assessment, Intervention, and Prevention*, 2nd ed. (Boston: Pearson, 2013), 4.

2. In H. Norman Wright, *The Complete Guide to Crisis and Trauma Counseling: What to Do and Say When It Matters Most* (Minneapolis, MN: Bethany House, 2011), there is a section on the crisis caused by the death

of a child. Wright at least mentions abortion: "When there is a miscarriage, stillbirth or infant death, it is called *the loss of possibility*. Children die because of abortion, kidnapping or running away" (286). He also includes a section titled "The Unrecognized Loss," which addresses the grief people experience alone because the loss is not recognized as a genuine loss by friends and family. The grief Wright has in immediate view is that arising from the death of a pet. Fortunately, a few people are acknowledging the hidden grief and trauma of abortion. See Theresa Burke, *Forbidden Grief: The Unspoken Pain of Abortion* (Springfield, IL: Acorn Books, 2002). See also, Michaelene Fredenberg, *Changed: Making Sense of Your Own or a Loved One's Abortion Experience* (San Diego, CA: Perspectives, 2008). For a distinctively Christian approach to abortion grief, see Patricia Layton, *Surrendering the Secret: Healing the Heartbreak of Abortion* (Nashville: Lifeway, 2008); and Kim Ketola, *Cradle My Heart: Finding God's Love after Abortion* (Grand Rapids: Kregel, 2012).

3. Burl E. Gilliland and Richard K. James, *Crisis Intervention Strategies*, 8th ed. (Boston: Cengage Learning, 2016).

4. On the history and formation of pregnancy crisis intervention services, see Peggy Hartshorn, *Foot Soldiers Armed with Love* (n.p.: Heartbeat International, 2014).

5. This is the number of pregnancy help offices that specialize in pregnancy crisis intervention listed in the Heartbeat International database of PHOs as of May 1, 2018. This figure does not include 403 safe homes for mothers, typically called Maternity Homes. But as they provide help to pregnant mothers, they certainly fit the definition of PHO. The total, then, would be 3,232.

6. Gilliland and James, 5.

7. See https://www.guttmacher.org/fact-sheet/induced-abortion-worldwide.

8. David C. Reardon, *Aborted Women, Silent No More* (Chicago: Loyola University Press, 1997), 10.

9. Frederica Mathewes-Green, *Real Choices: Listening to Women, Looking for Alternatives to Abortion* (Linthicum, MD: Felicity Press, 2013), 1.

10. "Facts on Induced Abortion in the United States," The Alan Guttmacher Institute (August 2011), http://www.guttmacher.org/pubs/bf_induced_abortion.html.

11. David Reardon, http://afterabortion.org/2004/rape-incest-and-abortion-searching-beyond-the-myths-3/.

12. Sandra K. Mahkorn, "Pregnancy and Sexual Assault," *The Psychological Aspects of Abortion*, ed. David Mall and Walter F. Watts (Washington, DC: University Publications of America, 1979), 55–69. David Reardon's study found a 73 percent birth rate among the 164 pregnant rape victims he interviewed. See David C. Reardon, Julie Makimaa, and Amy Sobie,

Victims and Victors: Speaking Out About Their Pregnancies, Abortions, and Children Resulting from Sexual Assault (Springfield, IL: Acorn Books, 2000).

13. For example, read Heather Gemmen's account of being raped at knifepoint, seeking out an abortion at first, but ultimately giving birth and parenting. *Startling Beauty: My Journey from Rape to Restoration* (Colorado Springs: Cook, 2004).

14. Gerald Caplan, *An Approach to Community Mental Health* (New York: Grune and Stratton, 1961), 18.

15. Douglas A. Puryear, *Helping People in Crisis* (San Francisco: Jossey-Bass, 1979), 6–7.

16. Mathewes-Green, 177.

17. Reardon, 11.

18. Ibid., 31.

19. Gilliland and James, 10.

20. See http://www.cincinnati.com/story/news/2015/12/12/abortion-cincinnati-the-most-important-decision-of-her-life/75948494/.

21. See http://www.cosmopolitan.com/politics/news/a54673/women-talk-about-why-they-had-an-abortion/.

22. See https://www.washingtonpost.com/opinions/im-a-successful-lawyer-and-mother-because-i-had-an-abortion/2016/01/22/d7dd75c6-c089-11e5-83d4-42e3bceea902_story.html. To clarify, she writes, "This quote, although not my own, explains why I joined my fellow lawyers in putting my name on this brief and sharing my story."

23. View the interview at http://www.pbs.org/wnet/tavissmiley/interviews/author-gloria-steinem/.

24. Wright, 162.

25. See Naomi Wolf, "Our Bodies, Our Souls," *The New Republic* (October 16, 1995): 26–35, https://lib.tcu.edu/staff/bellinger/abortion/Wolf-our-bodies.pdf.

Chapter 3

1. This understanding is so basic that one of the earliest and still commonly used training manuals for pregnancy crisis counseling is titled *The Love Approach*, written by Peggy Hartshorn and offered through Heartbeat International.

2. Jackson-Cherry and Erford, 56.

3. There are appropriate times and places to share these stories. Obtain permission from the woman or let her tell her own story in her own words. Within the context of a PHO, some women after the crisis are quite eager to share their story or let you tell it. Others will prefer ongoing privacy.

4. Jackson-Cherry and Erford, 51.

Chapter 4

1. Wendy Shalit, *A Return to Modesty: Discovering the Lost Virtue* (New York: Touchstone Books, 1999), 93.

2. Michaelene Fredenburg, *Changed* (San Diego, CA: Perspectives, 2013), 6–8. This account is taken from her booklet. She has a slightly altered version in her book *Changed: Making Sense of Your Own or a Loved One's Abortion Experience* (San Diego, CA: Perspectives, 2008), 25–31.

3. Wright, 21.

4. Andrew M. Coleman, *A Dictionary of Psychology*, 3d ed. (Oxford: Oxford University Press, 2008), http://oxfordindex.oup.com/view/10.1093/acref/9780199534067.013.2728. The concept of emotional intelligence as a cognitive ability is scientifically disputed. In counseling, most people refer to EI as a counseling tool or skill for understanding the presence and controlling influence of emotions. Since crisis as a human experience is primarily a state of emotional upheaval that disrupts normative cognitive abilities, EI is a helpful reference for crisis counseling.

5. We think of ourselves as in one mood or another. In reality, human beings are exceptionally complex in their emotions. Multiple emotions come as fast as differing thoughts. Observe, for example, the multiple emotions recorded in the event of Jesus healing a man with a withered hand in front of his religious opponents. "And he looked around at them with anger, grieved at their hardness of heart, and said to the man, 'Stretch out your hand.' He stretched it out, and his hand was restored" (Mark 3:5). Jesus was angry, grief-stricken, and compassionate at the same time. In this regard, he is fully human, just like us.

6. Scott Klusendorf, "Defending Your Prolife Views in Five Minutes or Less," in John Ensor and Scott Klusendorf, *Stand for Life* (Peabody, MA: Hendrickson Publishers, 2012), 8–11.

7. Fredenburg, *Changed*, 100–101.

8. Wright, 162.

9. Reardon, 10.

10. Fredenburg, *Changed* (2008), 101–2.

11. Shalit, 93.

12. I say "normally" to account for artificial reproductive technologies (ART).

13. Mathewes-Green, 124.

14. James and Gilliland, 42.

15. Ibid.

16. Ibid.

17. American Psychological Association, *Report of the Task Force on Mental Health and Abortion* (Washington, DC: APA, 2008), 11, http://www.apa.org/pi/wpo/mental-health-abortion-report.pdf.

Chapter 5

1. Priscilla Coleman, "Thirty Studies in Five Years Show Abortion Hurts Women's Mental Health," https://www.heartbeatinternational.org/30-studies-coleman.

2. *Salgo v. Leland Stanford Jr. University Board of Trustees* referenced in Ruth R. Faden and Tom L. Beauchamp, *A History and Theory of Informed Consent* (Oxford: Oxford University Press, 1986), 125.

3. *Making Health Care Decisions: The Ethical and Legal Implications of Informed Consent in the Patient-Practitioner Relationship* 3, no. 47 (1982), https://ia600403.us.archive.org/30/items/makinghealthcare00unit_1/makinghealthcare00unit_1.pdf.

4. *Making Health Care Decisions*, 65.

5. Maureen Paul, E. Steve Lichtenberg, Lynn Borgatta, David A. Grimes, Philip G. Stubblefield, and Mitchel D. Creinin, *Management of Unintended and Abnormal Pregnancy: Comprehensive Abortion Care* (Oxford: Wiley-Blackwell, 2009), 48 (emphasis original).

6. Canadian Medical Association, "CMA Code of Ethics" (2004), 2, https://www.cma.ca/Assets/assets-library/document/en/advocacy/policy-research/CMA_Policy_Code_of_ethics_of_the_Canadian_Medical_Association_Update_2004_PD04-06-e.pdf.

7. In explaining the science of MFA, I am indebted to the research collected and reviewed by Martha Shuping, MD.

8. J. T. Condon and C. Corkindale, "The Correlates of Antenatal Attachment in Pregnant Women," *British Journal of Medical Psychology* 70 (1997): 359–72.

9. "What Is Oxytocin?," *Psychology Today*, https://www.psychologytoday.com/basics/oxytocin.

10. S. Allanson and J. Astbury, "The Abortion Decision: Fantasy Processes," *Journal of Psychosomatic Obstetrics & Gynecology* (July 2009): 158–67, https://doi.org/10.3109/01674829609025677.

11. Maria Liljas Stålhandske, Marlene Makenzius, Tanja Tydén, and Margareta Larsson, "Existential Experiences and Needs Related to Induced Abortion in a Group of Swedish Women: A Quantitative Investigation," *Journal of Psychosomatic Obstetrics & Gynecology* (July 2011): 53–61, https://doi.org/10.3109/0167482X.2012.677877.

12. K. Dykes, P. Slade, and A. Haywood, "Long Term Follow-Up of Emotional Experiences after Termination of Pregnancy: Women's

Views at Menopause," *Journal of Reproductive and Infant Psychology* 29, no. 1 (2011): 1–20, https://doi.org/10.1080/02646838.2010.513046.

13. John C. Fletcher and Mark I. Evans, "Maternal Bonding in Early Fetal Ultrasound Examinations," *New England Journal of Medicine* (1983), 308:392-93, https://www.nejm.org/doi/full/10.1056/NEJM198302173080710.

14. PTS and PTSD refer to the same problem. Martha Shuping explains, "In 2013, the American Psychiatric Association published the 5th edition of its diagnostic manual, DSM-5, the most recent criteria for Posttraumatic Stress Disorder (PTSD). Many pertinent studies of PTSD used previous diagnostic criteria, but symptoms are similar. Many in the trauma field are removing the word 'disorder' and refer only to post-traumatic stress (PTS)." *Peace Psychology Perspectives on Abortion*, ed. Rachel M. MacNair (Kansas City, MO: Feminism & Nonviolence Studies Association, 2016), 154.

15. Personal correspondence, April 30, 2018.

16. A. Baker, T. Beresford, G. Halvorson-Boyd, and J. M. Garrity, "Informed Consent, Counseling, and Patient Preparation," in *A Clinician's Guide to Medical and Surgical Abortion*, ed. Maureen Paul, E. Steven Lichtenberg, Lynn Borgatta, David A. Grimes, and Phillip G. Stubblefield (Philadelphia, PA: Churchill Livingston, 1999), 28–29.

17. Angela Lanfranchi, Ian Gentles, and Elizabeth Ring-Cassidy, *Complications: Abortion's Impact on Women* (Toronto: The deVerber Institute of Bioethics and Social Research, 2013), 271–72.

18. Ibid., 273.

19. Erica Millar, *Happy Abortions: Our Bodies in the Era of Choice* (London: Zed Books, 2017), 278.

20. Ibid., 1. Millar expands, "The idea that women can have abortions so long as they feel 'really, really bad' about them balances the realization that abortion is necessary (and women will have them regardless of the legislative context) with concern for foetal life and the corresponding view that abortion is morally problematic. The 2015 Twitter campaign #ShoutYourAbortion was a direct response to cultural expectations about how women should approach and experience their abortion" (2).

21. Ibid., 157.

22. Brenda Major et al., Task Force on Mental Health and Abortion, *Report of the Task Force on Mental Health and Abortion* (Washington, DC: American Psychological Association 2008), 92, http://www.apa.org/pi/wpo/mental-health-abortion-report.pdf.

23. Martha Shuping, "Counterpoint: Long-Lasting Distress after Abortion," in *Peace Psychology Perspectives on Abortion*, 165.

24. Ibid., 166 (emphasis added).

25. Ibid., 167.

26. Lanfranchi et al., 255.

27. Ibid., 1 (emphasis original).

28. Priscilla K. Coleman, "Abortion and Mental Health: Quantitative Synthesis and Analysis of Research Published 1995–2009," *British Journal of Psychiatry* (2011): 119(3): 180–86.

29. Lanfranchi et al., 273.

30. Ibid., 274.

31. Ibid., 271.

32. Kathryn Dykes et al., "Long-Term Follow-Up of Emotional Experiences after Termination of Pregnancy: Women's Views at Menopause," *Journal of Reproductive and Infant Psychology* 29, no. 1 (2011), http://www.informaworld.com, DOI: 10.1080/02646838.2010.513046.

33. Paul et al., 57.

34. Ibid., 52–53.

35. Natalia Mufel, Anne Speckhard, and Sergei Sivuha, "Predictors of Posttraumatic Stress Disorder Following Abortion in a Former Soviet Union Country," *Journal of Prenatal and Perinatal Psych & Health* 17, no. 1 (Fall 2002): 50–51.

36. Baker et al., 27, 29.

37. For an index of studies, see Rachael MacNair, *Peace Psychology Perspectives on Abortion,* 29–35.

38. "Mandy's Testimony," in Martha Shuping, MFA, slides 78–80.

Chapter 6

1. Puryear, 51.

2. Wright, 164. The grief model can be found in Joanne T. Jozefowski, *The Phoenix Phenomenon: Rising from the Ashes of Grief* (Northvale, NJ: Jason Aronson, 1999).

3. George S. Everly, *Assisting Individuals in Crisis,* 5th ed. (Ellicott City, MD: International Critical Incident Foundation, 2015), 32–33.

4. Peggy Hartshorn, "The LOVE Approach," https://www.heartbeat international.org/pdf/TheLoveApproach.pdf.

5. Mathewes-Green, 23 (emphasis added).

6. Ibid., 12.

7. Reardon, *Aborted Women, Silent No More,* 35.

8. A positive pregnancy test verifies the presence of the hCG hormone, which is a leading indicator of pregnancy. However, other factors can create a false positive. Certain types of medication, hormone treatment, cancer, and even failure to use the test properly can lead to a positive result.

9. Censoring fetal development information from pregnant women is never justified. In abortion clinics, where there is a financial

gain in an abortion outcome, failure to disclose is a conflict of interest. Shielding a woman from a biological explanation of her pregnancy in the name of protecting her from discomfort violates the doctrine of informed consent (see chapter 5). A woman may decline the information or may choose to look away from the ultrasound screen. But ethically, informed consent is required for all medical procedures. It's the baseline for treating women with dignity.

10. Krissi Danielsson, "True Miscarriage Rates: Making Sense of Pregnancy Loss Statistics," http://miscarriage.about.com/od/pregnancy afterloss/qt/miscarriage-rates.htm.

11. Testifying to the complex and ambivalent feelings associated with pregnancy and abortion, some women, intending to abort, will nonetheless become visibly upset and express grief upon discovery of a fetal demise or early stage miscarriage.

12. *US Food and Drug Administration Medication Guide: Mifeprex* (2011), http://www.fda.gov/downloads/drugs/drugsafety/postmarketdrug safetyinformationforpatientsandproviders/ucm258412.pdf.

13. "Choices," Life Choices Health Network, http://lifechoices.org.

14. Wright, 21.

Chapter 7

1. R.P. Bedi, "Concept Mapping the Client's Perspective on Counseling Alliance Formation," *Journal of Counseling Psychology* 53 (2006): 26–35. The quote comes from Jackson-Cherry and Erford, 68.

2. Jackson-Cherry and Erford, 70.

3. Fredenburg, 8.

4. Ibid., 37.